CLINICAL USE OF ANTICONVULSANTS
IN PSYCHIATRIC DISORDERS

Clinical Use of Anticonvulsants in Psychiatric Disorders

Robert M. Post, M.D.

Chief, Biological Psychiatry Branch
National Institute of Mental Health
Chevy Chase, Maryland

Michael R. Trimble, F.R.C.P., F.R.C. (Psych)

Consultant Physician and
Raymond-Way Senior Lecturer
Department of Neurology
Institute of Neurology
London, England

C.E. Pippenger, Ph.D.

Head, Section of Applied Clinical Pharmacology
Department of Biochemistry
The Cleveland Clinic Foundation
Cleveland, Ohio

Demos Publications, 156 Fifth Avenue, New York, New York 10010

© 1989 by Demos Publications Inc. All rights reserved. This book is protected by copyright. No part of it may be reproduced, stored in a retrieval system, or transmitted in any form or by any means, electronic, mechanical, photocopying, recording, or otherwise, without the prior written permission of the publisher.

Made in the United States of America

ISBN: 0-939957-20-5
LC: 89-050472

Preface

In recent years there has been a growing interest in the use of anticonvulsant drugs for conditions other than epilepsy. For example, carbamazepine is considered a drug of choice for the treatment of trigeminal neuralgia and related paroxysmal pain syndromes. The value of anticonvulsants in the treatment of some psychiatric disorders is also increasingly recognized. Historically, there has been considerable use of anticonvulsant agents in the treatment of neuropsychiatric patients. Bromides were widely prescribed in the last century, barbiturates in the early part of this century, and more recently there has been extensive use of benzodiazepines. These drugs are effective anticonvulsants, but their clinical use in psychiatry has been restricted to their consideration as sedatives, hypnotics, or minor tranquilizers. In the midpart of the century, psychiatry widely used the seizures of electroconvulsive therapy for treatment of the mood disorders. In retrospect, it now appears that this somatic treatment conveys potent anticonvulsant properties and is perhaps the first widely used anticonvulsant treatment for the major affective disorders. Most recently, carbamazepine and valproic acid have emerged as additional treatment options for the lithium-refractory bipolar patient.

The history of carbamazepine is of interest, as the compound was first synthesized for its possible antidepressant properties but discounted for this indication because of its unusual behavioral pharmacological profile. Its anticonvulsant and antinociceptive properties were then recognized and carbamazepine was introduced in Europe for the management of epilepsy in the early 1960s. By the early and mid-1970s, extensive reports suggested that it had "psychotropic" properties in this patient population. These data, as well as its ability to stabilize limbic system excitability, led to the first controlled trials of carbamazepine in the United States and, later, several European countries. Earlier uncontrolled studies had been performed in Japan, suggesting its value in bipolar affective disorder. These data and reports of the possible value of carbamazepine in other conditions, such as episodic dyscontrol and as an adjunct to neuroleptics in schizophrenia, led to a wider series of investigations and to studies of other anticonvulsant agents such as valproic acid and clonazepam in the affective and related disorders.

There are now a growing number of studies evaluating the use of a variety of anticonvulsants in several neuropsychiatric conditions. As a consequence, many of these agents have become part of the armamentarium of the practicing psychiatrist as well as neurologists interested in potential psychotropic effects of these agents. However, because of the rapidly emerging data base in this area, many physicians are not well acquainted with this class of anticonvulsant compounds, their dose schedules, side effects, and pharmacokinetic profiles. For this reason, this book has been written in the hope that it will be a practical guide to anticonvulsant use for those seeking such knowledge. It is aimed at providing practical information for the clinician. It is meant to integrate both an extensive literature in this area and our own practical clinical experience with the anticonvulsant drugs in a variety of neuropsychiatric disorders.

Two chapters are devoted to the use of these compounds in the treatment of epileptic patients and to discussion of the interfaces between epilepsy and psychiatry. Three chapters provide basic information about the anticonvulsant drugs, their chemistry, pharmacokinetics, and general principles regarding their prescription. The major focus of the book is on the use of anticonvulsants in clinical psychiatric syndromes. This includes both areas in which there is wide recognition of the value of the anticonvulsants, such as in bipolar illness, as well as preliminary areas that are still in the process of evaluation, such as the use of these compounds in episodic dyscontrol, schizoaffective and schizophrenic disorders. A section is also included on childhood disorders.

We hope this text will be of value to a wide range of practitioners who wish to expand the potential of the anticonvulsants as psychotropic agents. As such, it continues to explore one interface between neurology and psychiatry; namely, how the use of antiepileptic drugs may further elucidate the robust and, at times, subtle and complicated interrelationships between seizures and psychiatric disorders.

R.M.P., M.R.T., and C.E.P.
1989

Contents

1. Epilepsy and Its Classification   1

2. Psychiatric Problems in Epilepsy and Their Management   17

3. Principles of Applied Clinical Pharmacology: A Guide to Therapeutics   41

4. Clinically Significant Antiepileptic Drug Interactions   71

5. Pharmacodynamics of Antiepileptic Drugs   89

6. Behavioral Disorders in Childhood   99

7. Use of Anticonvulsants in the Treatment of Manic-Depressive Illness   113

8. Anticonvulsants as Adjuncts to Neuroleptics in the Treatment of Schizoaffective and Schizophrenic Patients   153

9. Anticonvulsants in the Treatment of Aggression and Dyscontrol   165

Index   177

1

Epilepsy and Its Classification

Michael R. Trimble

Full consideration of the rational use of antiepileptic drugs in psychiatry requires an understanding of their use in epilepsy, and further consideration of the relationship between epilepsy and psychiatry. Although to many the term epilepsy appears to be one without controversy, in reality its definition is as easy or as difficult as that of some psychiatric conditions such as schizophrenia. Hughlings Jackson gave the often-quoted definition that epilepsy was "an occasional, sudden, rapid and local discharge of grey matter," but this essentially defines the seizure, and emphasizes the acute paroxysmal nature of the condition. However, this definition fails to distinguish epilepsy from other similar disorders (e.g., migraines or acute panic attacks, or even a sneeze). It is accepted that any definition of epilepsy requires recurrent as opposed to single seizures, and recognizes that epilepsy is a heterogeneous group of conditions. Perhaps, as Bleuler renamed dementia precox "the schizophrenias," it is most appropriate to refer to "the epilepsies." As with schizophrenia, clear evidence for organic brain dysfunction becomes more evident the more it is looked for, but in a number of cases, even with modern technology, recurrent seizures are found in the absence of identifiable neuropathology.

Epilepsy is then the tendency to have recurrent seizures, and can be diagnosed once that tendency has been expressed. It is not uncommon in psychiatric practice to meet patients who have isolated seizures, and as such, these patients should not be diagnosed as epileptics. Good examples are seizures occurring following withdrawal from alcohol or benzodiazepines, or the occasional seizure precipitated by the administration of tricyclic drugs or neuroleptic drugs, particularly to patients who have a lower seizure threshold. A list of drugs used in psychiatric practice likely to lower the seizure threshold is shown in Table 1-1.

CLASSIFICATION

It is important to distinguish the classification of seizures from the classification of epilepsy. Recently, several classifications of seizures have

Table 1-1. Drugs Used in Psychiatry Likely to Lower the Seizure Threshold

Antidepressants: Particularly tricyclic drugs, especially mianserin, maprotiline
Major tranquilizers: Phenothiazines, especially chlorpromazine

emerged and an abbreviated version of the latest one is shown in Table 1-2.

This classification essentially divides seizures into those which arise focally, within some identifiable region of the brain referred to as partial seizures, and those where no focal onset can be discerned referred to as generalized seizures. Partial seizures are those in which the clinical findings and the EEG changes clarify that the onset arises from a focus, and the subsequent breakdown of the seizure type then depends upon whether or not consciousness is impaired during the attack. In simple partial seizures, consciousness is retained. Various forms are recognized (e.g., focal motor seizures [when accompanied by a spreading "march" of motor involvement these are referred to as jacksonian]); with somatosensory or special sensory symptoms; with autonomic symptoms; or associated with psychic symptoms such as dysphasia, dysmnesia (e.g., deja vu), or cognitive, affective, illusory, or hallucinatory experiences. In general, this last group of symptoms is usually accompanied by impairment of consciousness and, when occurring in epilepsy, is usually associated with the diagnosis of complex partial seizure. In the latter, impairment of consciousness is often the first clinical sign, although simple partial seizures may evolve into the complex variety. In patients presenting to psychiatric clinics, complex partial seizures are the most common seizure type. Patients usually, but not inevitably, will give a history of a progression from complex partial seizures to a secondary generalized motor seizure on some occasions.

Generalized seizures are those in which the first clinical changes suggest

Table 1-2. Revised International League Against Epilepsy (ILAE) Classification of Epileptic Seizures

I. Partial (focal, local) seizures
   A. Simple partial seizures (consciousness not impaired)
   B. Complex partial seizures (with impairment of consciousness: may sometimes begin with simple symptomatology)
   C. Partial seizures evolving to secondarily generalized seizures (this may be generalized tonic-clonic, tonic, or clonic)
II. Generalized seizures (convulsive or nonconvulsive)
III. Unclassified epileptic seizure

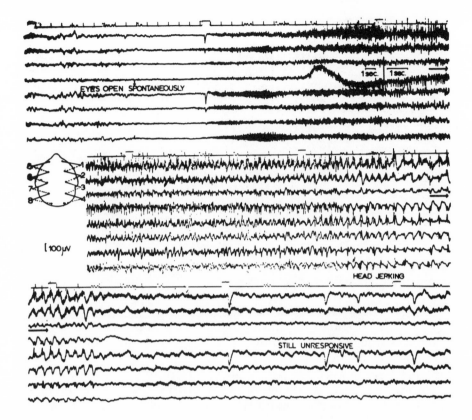

FIG. 1-1. The EEG of a generalized tonic-clonic seizure. This shows some pre-ictal flattening of the record. Note the postictal slow waves.

bilateral abnormalities with widespread disturbances in both hemispheres (Fig. 1-1). Absence seizures (petit mal) are usually associated with regular 3 Hz/second spike and slow wave activity on the EEG, although variants of this with 2–3 Hz activity may be seen (Fig. 1-2).

Myoclonic seizures typically present with myoclonic jerking, and these are sometimes associated with clearly delineated EEG changes. Tonic-clonic seizures are the classical grand mal attacks with associated EEG abnormalities. They are clinically unmistakable. There is a sudden loss of consciousness, often without warning, and tonic muscular contractions are followed by clonic ones. The patient falls to the ground, during which time self-injury may occur and tongue biting or urinary incontinence may be noted. Following the attack, the patient is unrousable for a time and there may be a period of postictal confusion. If the attack has a focal origin prior to its generalization, then the patient may report an aura, namely a brief feeling or sensation immediately before the attack which

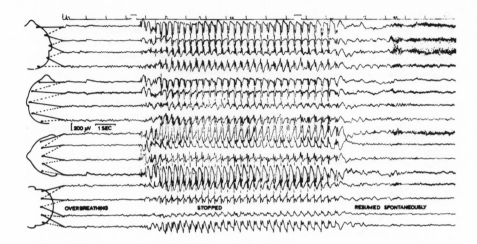

FIG. 1-2. The EEG of classical petit mal epilepsy with 3/second spike wave activity. During the abnormality the patient is unresponsive.

represents the origin of the epileptic activity. If this proceeds no further, it would be a simple partial seizure. These auras need to be distinguished from prodromata, which occur several hours or even days before a seizure and serve to warn the patient about a forthcoming seizure. Prodromal symptoms are of great interest to psychiatrists because they often involve changes of mood, in particular dysphoria and irritability. They may also present as headaches or changes of appetite.

Generalized seizures presenting as absence attacks impair consciousness briefly, and are virtually unaccompanied by motor signs. Brief flickering of the eyelids is usually all that is noted, and if patients have more obvious or prolonged motor manifestations with brief epileptic seizures, it is more likely that they are having a focal seizure. Generalized absence seizures occur primarily in children, and in many cases, cease before the age of 20. In approximately 50% of patients this form of seizure is replaced by a generalized tonic-clonic seizure. The most disruptive feature of the generalized absence seizure is the amnesia for the moments of the attack which, if occurring many times a day, can be disruptive to educational and vocational activities.

Partial Seizures

The symptoms of focal attacks correspond to the site of origin of the abnormal electrical activity in the brain, and the most common disturbances seen in psychiatric practice relate to a temporal lobe location. There may be disturbance of thought, perception, behavior, affect, and in complex partial seizures, consciousness. Hallucinations may be formed and complex, as opposed to those that arise from seizures of primary sensory cortex which are usually simple (e.g., flashes of light). Characteristically in epilepsy, the hallucination is constant, very vivid, and with repeated episodes is carefully reproduced. Any recognized emotion may occur, although the most common experience is fear, which is intense, vivid, and may be associated with fear of death. The paroxysmal nature of this episodic fear and its quality are highly reminiscent of panic attacks and patients with panic disorder are often misdiagnosed as having epilepsy, and vice versa.

Depression is an uncommon but well-documented ictal symptom, although rage and outbursts of anger are rare. Nonetheless, given the right environment, it is clear that directed anger can occur as the result of an ictus, and this has important forensic implications.

Cursive seizures refer to running attacks; gelastic seizures are laughing attacks. In uncinate seizures, the patient experiences an unpleasant smell or taste, and this may be accompanied by chewing movements and lip smacking.

Myoclonic seizures are sudden, brief, jerk-like contractions which may be generalized or confined to one or more muscle groups. They may be solitary or repetitive and may be triggered by actions. They commonly occur late at night or early in the morning and, in some people, herald a generalized tonic-clonic seizure.

Automatisms, which may occur with partial or generalized seizures, refer to all kinds of motor and behavior acts that occur within the peri-ictal period. They are usually associated with the immediate postictal period, but clearly in some patients, the abnormalities of behavior begin as part of the ictus. In many they may be very slight and just be brief lip smacking and abnormal posturing, while occasionally, particularly if prolonged, they may present as severely disruptive behavior leading to self or other injury. Characteristically, the motor activity is automatic and occurs during a state of altered consciousness. There is usually total amnesia for the episode, although as time passes and the automatism wanes, the environment begins to have more of an influence over the patient's behavior and the amnesia may only be partial. Automatisms may be either perseverative, in which patients continue to do actions they were involved in prior to the attack, or they may herald the initiative of a completely new behavioral sequence. The neurophysiological basis for automatism is thought to be bilateral involvement of the amygdaloid-hippocampal region of the limbic system.

Status epilepticus denotes recurrent epileptic seizures without return of consciousness between attacks. Persistent focal seizures are referred to as epilepsia partialis continua and when complex partial seizures are continuous, the condition complex partial seizure status is diagnosed. These may be associated with prolonged states of behavior disturbance occurring with minimal alteration of higher cognitive function. The associated hallucinations and delusions closely resemble psychiatric conditions (e.g., an affective disorder or a schizophrenia). The following two case histories are representative.

Case One

A 22-year-old right-handed housewife presented with feelings of uneasiness for 9 months and bouts of depression for 4 years. Two aunts in the family had been treated for depression. For 6 to 9 months prior to the presentation, she complained of headaches, things appearing distant, and a subjective feeling of uneasiness with "butterflies in the stomach." She became increasingly depressed with excessive tiredness, crying, loss of appetite, weight, and libido, loss of interest in things, and early morning wakening. She had experienced "attacks" during which her husband reported that she "cringed," her arms flexed, she shuddered and shouted. These attacks lasted 15–20 seconds, followed by drowsiness for a further 15–20 seconds. She had these episodes from one to four times a day. An EEG showed continuous high-voltage epileptic discharges from the right anterior temporal region amounting to a temporal lobe status. She was commenced on carbamazepine in increasing doses, the EEG normalized and the patient became asymptomatic with no further attacks of depression.

Case Two

A 22-year-old man, with a history of complex partial and generalized tonic-clonic seizures since the age of 3½, had the sudden onset of "indescribable feelings" that rays were being passed through his body in order to sterilize him. Subsequently he heard voices criticizing him in both the second and third persons and was admitted to a psychiatric hospital with an acute psychosis, diagnosed as schizophrenia.

While under observation, his mental state was variable, at times being torpid and hardly responsive, at other times restless and demanding to go home. As he became communicative, it was clear he had a florid paranoid psychosis with schizophreniform features. An EEG was carried out, showing frequent sharp waves on the right side with phase reversals at the right sphenoidal electrode which were almost continuous (Fig. 1-3).

The patient's mental state responded promptly to intravenous diazepam, as did the electroencephalographic disturbance. Over the ensuing months he was readmitted to a mental hospital on several occasions with acute onset episodes of a similar psychosis.

Summary

In contrast, during absence status, prolonged alteration of cognitive function occurs with intermittent prolonged stupor. This, too, may occa-

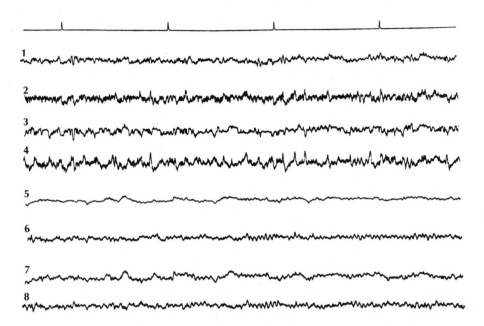

FIG. 1-3. The EEG of case 2 showing continuous high voltage epileptic discharges from the right anterior temporal region. The electrodes are as follows: **(1)**, Fp2-F8; **(2)**, F8-T4; **(3)**, Fp2-R sphenoidal; **(4)**, R sphenoidal-T4; **(5)**, Fp1-F7; **(6)**, F7-T3; **(7)**, Fp1-L sphenoidal; **(8)**, L sphenoidal-T3. Note the frequent sharp waves on the right with phase reversal at the right sphenoidal electrodes.

sionally present as a psychotic illness, with hallucinations and delusions intermingled with a fluctuating confusional state and the associated EEG changes.

CLASSIFICATION OF THE EPILEPSIES

In contrast to the classification of seizures which has now gone through several editions, the classification of the epilepsies has proved much more difficult. A provisional classification has recently been published and is shown in Table 1-3. This is essentially a classification of syndromes rather than diseases, and, as with classification in psychiatry, the consensus of opinion as to the most appropriate way to classify the epilepsies has yet to be reached.

Terms used by earlier versions of classifications, such as primary and secondary, have been omitted, and the main dichotomy separates epilepsies with generalized seizures from those with partial or focal seizures, the latter being referred to as localization-related partial or focal epilepsies. Of particular relevance for psychiatrists are the localization-related symp-

Table 1-3. ILAE Classification of Epilepsies

---

1. Localization-related (focal, local, partial) epilepsies and syndromes
   Idiopathic with age-related onset (e.g., benign epilepsy of childhood)
   Symptomatic (e.g., frontal lobe, temporal lobe)
2. Generalized epilepsies or syndromes
   Idiopathic
   Idiopathic and/or symptomatic (e.g., West's syndrome)
   Symptomatic
3. Epilepsies and syndromes undetermined as to whether they are focal or generalized
4. Special syndromes (e.g., febrile convulsions)

---

tomatic seizures, further designated by the area of localization affected. For example, frontal lobe epilepsies often present as brief episodes of behavior change with minimal or no postictal confusion. There may be deviation of the head and eyes, sometimes referred to as an adversive seizure. Nonetheless, the frontal lobe epilepsies can present with florid episodes of bizarre behavior, which on occasion may be mistaken for hysteria.

Under temporal lobe epilepsies there is a category of limbic epilepsies, with particular emphasis on hippocampal and amygdala pathology. These epilepsies characteristically present with partial seizures, alteration of consciousness, and often automatisms.

Some distinctive syndromes included in the classification of the epilepsies should be mentioned. West's syndrome (infantile spasms) consists of a characteristic picture of infantile spasms in association with hypsarrhythmia on the EEG. The onset is in the first year of life, and the spasms are flexor or extensor or both. The importance of the syndrome is that it is not uncommonly associated with the later development of mental retardation. The Lennox-Gastaut syndrome occurs in children up to the age of about 8, and presents with a variety of attacks, focal, myoclonic, atonic, and absence, with a markedly disturbed EEG and associated mental retardation.

THE CAUSES OF EPILEPSY

Some underlying pathologies and metabolic defects related to seizures in epilepsy are outlined in Table 1-4. There is variation with age, neonatal seizures being caused by prenatal events such as cerebral malformations, rubella embryopathy, toxoplasmosis, and perinatal birth damage from hypoxia or trauma. Postnatal events include metabolic changes such as hypoglycemia, hypocalcemia, hypomagnesemia, infections such as meningi-

Table 1-4. Some Causes of Epilepsy

Category	Cause
Metabolic	Hypoglycemia, hypomagnesemia, fluid and electrolyte disturbances, acute intermittent porphyria, amino acid disorders
Trauma	Head injuries, especially penetrating wounds and birth injuries
Neurological	Tumors, cerebrovascular accidents, degenerative and storage disorders, demyelinating diseases, Sturge-Weber and other malformations, tuberous sclerosis, infections (e.g., cytomegalovirus, toxoplasmosis, meningitis, cysticercosis, syphilis)
Drug withdrawal	Especially alcohol and barbiturates
Vitamin deficiency	Pyridoxine
Poisons	Lead, strychnine
Temperature	Fever

tis, and a number of inborn errors of metabolism which become expressed early in life.

Early childhood epilepsy (starting around the age of 3) is more likely to be idiopathic, whereas in adult life, tumors and cerebrovascular diseases become prominent causes. Head injury is common at any age, and is most likely to occur if during the injury the dura is penetrated or if there is coma and a posttraumatic amnesia of more than 24 hours. Early seizures following injury increases the probability of later development of epilepsy, and the pattern is usually that of focal or secondary generalized attacks. Fifty percent of patients who develop posttraumatic epilepsy have their first attack within 12 months of the injury, although in some cases the onset may be delayed for several years. Posttraumatic psychosis following head injury is very often associated with the development of seizures.

Why patients have seizures when they do is not clear, although reflex epilepsy, where seizures are provoked by sensory or motor events, has been well described. Visually evoked seizures, by photic stimulation and musicogenic seizures, in which attacks are triggered by patterned tones are well-known examples. "Psychogenic seizures," where seizures are evoked by specific mental activity, also occur. In these, a direct act of the will may precipitate a seizure (e.g., intense concentration or sudden alteration of attention). Alternatively, a seizure may be precipitated by a mental act without the deliberate intention of the patient. This might include attacks brought on by mental arithmetic. The term *psychogenic seizure* is more appropriately reserved for these kinds of episodes, in which some clearly defined mental event precipitates the seizure. It is often, mistakenly, used for seizures that are nonepileptic in origin, perhaps more commonly referred to as *pseudoseizures.*

EPILEPSY AND THE USE OF ANTIEPILEPTIC DRUGS

In general, the older barbiturate-related compounds and phenytoin are being replaced by the newer drugs such as carbamazepine and valproic acid. One of the problems with the older drugs has been the growing recognition of chronic toxic side effects that occur with the long-term administration that the treatment of epilepsy obviously requires. Table 1-5 gives a list of the commonly used anticonvulsant drugs and the seizures that they are usually used to control. Some important facts should be noted. First, some drugs are very specific, e.g., ethosuximide, which is only of value in generalized absence seizures. The more the EEG pattern conforms to the typical 3 Hz/second spike wave type, the more likely is the response. Secondly, carbamazepine is of no value in generalized absence seizures, and neither is it helpful for the prevention of febrile seizures in childhood.

As can be seen from the list, most of the drugs cover a fairly wide spectrum of activity, being of value against simple and complex partial seizures, generalized tonic-clonic seizures, and secondary generalized seizures. The drug of choice for partial seizures is carbamazepine. Its superiority over other anticonvulsants in this condition is now being recognized. It is also of value for the treatment of simple partial seizures and

Table 1-5. Some Anticonvulsant Drugs in Current Use

Name	Indications
Carbamazepine (Tegretol) Clobazam (Frisium)	Generalized seizures; simple or complex partial seizures; secondary generalized seizures
Clonazepam (Rivotril, Klonopin)	Myoclonic epilepsy
Ethosuximide (Zarotin)	Generalized absence seizures
Phenobarbitone	Generalized or simple partial seizures
Phenytoin (Epanutin, Dilantin)	Generalized seizures: simple or complex partial seizures
Primidone (Mysoline)	Generalized: complex or simple partial seizures
Valproic acid (Epilim, Depakene)	Generalized absence seizures: myoclonic epilepsy; simple or complex partial seizures
Sulthiame (Ospolot)	Complex partial seizures

generalized seizures. Valproic acid is commonly used to treat generalized absence seizures, and is of value in generalized tonic-clonic and myoclonic seizures. It is less widely used for simple or complex partial seizures. Phenytoin has a wide spectrum of activity, but side effects (see below) limit its usefulness. The same would be said for phenobarbitone. Finally, some benzodiazepine drugs such as clonazepam, nitrazepam, and more recently clobazam, have been used in a variety of seizure types, particularly difficult to control partial seizures and generalized and myoclonic seizures.

SIDE EFFECTS OF ANTICONVULSANTS

Acute toxic effects have been recognized for a long time, and include such obvious problems as nausea, vomiting, ataxia, dizziness, vertigo, headache, disorientation, and a variety of subjective phenomena. However, it is the chronic ones which especially include changes of cognitive function and behavior that are of particular importance to psychiatry. Further, interactions between anticonvulsants as discussed in Chapter 4 may present problems, as may interactions with psychotropic drugs. The chronic toxic effects are shown in Table 1-6.

Neuropsychiatric side effects, in particular those from phenytoin, include an encephalopathy and deterioration of intellectual function, whereas apathy, depression, dysphoria, irritability, and occasionally hyperactivity are seen in association with barbiturates and polytherapy. Chronic dyskinesias are occasionally seen, although an acute dystonic reaction has been noted with carbamazepine. Idiosyncratic psychotic reactions have been described with carbamazepine, ethosuximide, phenytoin, and primidone.

In recent years it has become clear that anticonvulsant drugs themselves have an important influence on cognitive abilities. For most anticonvulsants, detrimental effects on neuropsychological abilities have now been reported, although the nature of the deficits tends to vary between the studies. Generally they are such that they might be expected to interfere, at least with an individual's capacity to function at his peak efficiency at work, at school, and in other daily activities. As a generalization, phenobarbitone is the drug most implicated, carbamazepine the least. Another finding that is emerging from more recent studies is that a relationship between anticonvulsant serum concentrations and cognitive functioning, with high but not necessarily toxic levels, is associated with neuropsychological impairment. Thus, the acceptance of an upper limit of tolerance has relevance with regard to the more gross aspects of neuropsychiatric impairment provoked by these drugs, but subtle changes, especially those of cognitive function, are now known to occur within the tolerance limits. Further, they probably do not occur idiosyncratically, but are seen in all people, irrespective of whether they have epilepsy or not.

Table 1-6. Chronic Toxic Effects of Some Anticonvulsant Drugs

Nervous system	Cerebellar atrophy (?)
	Peripheral neuropathy
	Encephalopathy
	Other mental symptoms
Hemopoietic system	Folic acid deficiency
	Neonatal coagulation defects
Skeletal system	Metabolic bone disease
	Vitamin D deficiency
Connective tissue	Gum hypertrophy
	Facial skin changes
	Wound healing
	Dupuytren's contracture
Skin	Hirsutism
	Pigmentation
	Acne
Liver	Enzyme induction
Endocrine system	Pituitary-adrenal
	Thyroid-parathyroid
	Hyperglycemia (diabetogenic)
Other metabolic disorders	Vitamin B_6 deficiency (?)
	Heavy metals
Immunological disorders	Lymphotoxicity
	Lymphadenopathy
	Systemic lupus erythematosus
	Antinuclear antibodies
	Immunoglobulin changes (?)
	Immunosuppression

A series of studies has been conducted to assess the kind of impairments that anticonvulsant drugs may provoke and the differences between individual drugs. Trimble and colleagues examined several anticonvulsants including phenytoin, carbamazepine, sodium valproate, clobazam, and clonazepam in both patients and in double-blind controlled studies of volunteers who did not suffer from epilepsy. Significant deficits in performance were recorded for all five of these drugs. Impairments were most marked following phenytoin, and occurred on measures of memory, mental, and motor speed. These recorded deficits were observed at mean anticonvulsant levels within the so-called therapeutic range. Furthermore, significant correlations were observed between individual serum levels and the degree of deterioration in test performance on several measures (Figs. 1-4 and 1-5). Following clonazepam, at the modest dose of 0.5 mg three times daily, impairments of memory and coding tasks were found. However, deficits were fewer with sodium valproate,

Significant Differences Between the High and Low Serum Level Sessions

	DPH	NaV	CBZ
MEMORY			
Pictures:			
Immediate recall	●	●	
CONCENTRATION			
Stroop:			
Naming speed			●
Visual scanning:			
Alone		●	
With auditory task	●	●	
Auditory task:			
Part 3	●	●	
MENTAL SPEED			
Decision making:			
Category	●	●	
MOTOR SPEED			
Tapping:			
Dominant hand	●		
Both			●

● p at least <0.05

FIG. 1-4. Significant impairments in patients on higher levels of anticonvulsants. DPH, phenytoin; NaV, valproic acid; CBZ, carbamazepine.

carbamazepine, and clobazam. With sodium valproate and clobazam, the pattern suggested a slowing down of mental processing speed, which reached significance only when the demands of the task increased. In contrast, those in association with carbamazepine occurred in relation to motor rather than cognitive speed, and did not appear to significantly influ-

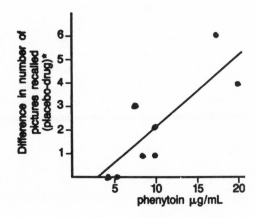

FIG. 1-5. Relationship between phenytoin serum levels and memory impairment in a study of picture recall is shown. In these eight volunteers, the higher the serum level of phenytoin, the greater the difference in picture recall versus placebo. *The higher the score, the greater the impairment. (From Thompson and Trimble, unpublished observations.)

Table 1-7.   Behavioral Toxicity of Anticonvulsant Drugs' Effects on Cognitive Function

Drugs	Patients	Volunteers
Carbamazepine	Minimal	Minimal
Clobazam	Minimal	Minimal
Clonazepam	Impairs	Impairs
Ethosuximide	Variable	Not tested
Phenobarbitone	Impairs	Impairs
Phenytoin	Impairs	Impairs
Valproic acid	Mild impairment	Minimal

ence higher cognitive function. Interestingly, on one test of processing speed, perceptual registration, the speed at which a sensory stimulus could be recognized, was improved on carbamazepine.

In studies with patients, changes in performance have been noted following medication changes. The overall findings are that drug reductions in patients on polytherapy improve performance on psychological tests, the improvements occurring across a wide spectrum of cognitive abilities. Improvements are most marked on measures of concentration and motor speed, and least marked on measures of memory. These observed benefits were generally not seen to be significant until 3 to 6 months following the drug changes, suggesting that some time may need to elapse before it is advisable to evaluate the consequences of drug manipulations on cognitive abilities. Improvements in neuropsychological functioning often take place in the absence of any marked changes in seizure frequency, although one of the benefits of drug reductions in such patients may be an improvement in seizure control.

Table 1-7 summarizes the data from several studies of these kinds of investigations, showing a spectrum of the behavioral toxicity of anticonvulsant drugs in relationship to intellectual function.

Valproic acid has been associated with liver failure in a small number of young patients, particularly in mentally handicapped children receiving multiple drugs. It may also produce a reversible alopecia and weight gain. Carbamazepine may be associated with water intoxication, although the mechanism of this is not clear. However, some patients present with hyponatremia and low osmolality while on carbamazepine, which paradoxically may also be linked with psychogenic polydipsia. This leads to a confusing clinical picture, but the problem may resolve on withdrawal of the carbamazepine. This incidentally is in contrast to the polyuria provoked by lithium and emphasizes the different pharmacological profiles of lithium and carbamazepine, although both have mood-stabilizing effects (see Chapter 7).

A paradoxical effect of the antiepileptic drugs is that they may increase seizures. Thus, like many drugs in medicine, they may have a biphasic action. While being anticonvulsant within a certain therapeutic range, at high levels they may provoke seizures. This appears to be exacerbated by multiple drug therapy. Thus, although it is now generally accepted that newly diagnosed patients should be treated by the prescription of only one anticonvulsant drug if possible, many patients still receive polytherapy. It has been shown that upwards of 80% of new patients, adults or children, if appropriate serum level monitoring is used to assess anticonvulsant levels, and adequate serum levels are achieved, can be satisfactorily controlled with one drug alone. Although there are obviously some patients who require a second drug (e.g., those with two different seizure types responding to different drugs) it has yet to be clearly demonstrated that generally the addition of a second drug leads to better management of seizures than the use of one drug. The use of polytherapy is not an uncommon situation in psychiatry where a patient may be receiving two or three benzodiazepines, one or two anticonvulsants, or two or three neuroleptic drugs, where one drug of each group may suffice. In epilepsy, a number of trials have been carried out in which patients receiving polytherapy had their therapy rationalized so that they are receiving monotherapy. This often brings with it an improvement in the seizure frequency, but also lessens the side effects that patients have, most notably the behavior and cognitive ones.

For patients with psychiatric disabilities, both phenobarbitone and phenytoin are unsuitable as noted. Phenytoin is a particularly difficult drug for patients where compliance may be at issue because of its unstable pharmacokinetics (see Chapter 3), but it also includes among its side effects hirsutism, gum hypertrophy, acne, and coarsening of the facial features. These secondary effects are liable to increase the psychosocial problems of patients with epilepsy further, especially if they are female. Another reason not to prescribe phenytoin for female patients of child-bearing age is the interaction with the contraceptive pill which may lead to unwanted pregnancy, and the teratogenic effects which have been established for this and several anticonvulsant drugs, being probably minimal with carbamazepine.

Generally, doses of the anticonvulsant drug prescribed will vary with each individual, although it is wise to start with a small dose and increase gradually until satisfactory serum levels have been achieved. Thus, one of the great advances in the management of epilepsy in recent years has been the introduction of serum level monitoring to tailor the patient's dosage to their own metabolic requirements. Where possible, anticonvulsants should be given on a once or twice daily regime, although with several of the anticonvulsant drugs as noted, this cannot be done. However, in patients where compliance is a problem, the minimum number of prescriptions daily should be tried.

SUGGESTED READING

Delgado-Escueta A, Mattson R, King L. The nature of aggression during epileptic seizures. *N Engl J Med* 1981;305:711–716.

Fenwick P. Precipitation and inhibition of seizures. In: Reynolds EH, Trimble MR, eds. *Epilepsy and Psychiatry*. Edinburgh: Churchill Livingstone, 1981:242–263.

International League Against Epilepsy. Proposal for revised clinical and electroencephalographic classification of epileptic seizures. *Epilepsia* 1981;22:489–501.

International League Against Epilepsy. Proposal for classification of the epilepsies and epileptic syndromes. *Epilepsia* 1985;26:268–278.

Laidlaw J, Richens A, Oxley J. *A Textbook of Epilepsy*, 3rd ed. Edinburgh: Churchill Livingstone, 1987.

Mattson RH, Cramer JA, Collins JF, VA Group. Comparison of carbamazepine, phenobarbitol, phenytoin and primidone in partial and secondarily generalized tonic-clonic seizures. *N Engl J Med* 1985;313:145–151

Reynolds EH. Chronic antiepileptic toxicity review. *Epilepsia* 1975;16:319–352.

Thompson PJ, Trimble MR. Anticonvulsant drugs and cognitive function. *Epilepsia* 1982;23:531–544.

Thompson PJ, Trimble MR. Sodium valproate and cognitive function in normal volunteers. *Br J Clin Pharmacol* 1981;12:819–824.

Thompson PJ, Trimble MR. Clobazam and cognitive function: effects on healthy volunteers. In: *Royal Society of Medicine International Congress and Symposium Series*. London: Academic Press, 1981:33–38.

Trimble MR, Reynolds EH. Neuropsychiatric toxicity of anticonvulsant drugs. In: Matthews B, ed. *Recent Advances in Neurology*. Edinburgh: Churchill Livingstone, 1984:261–280.

Trimble MR, Reynolds EH. *What Is Epilepsy?* Edinburgh: Churchill Livingstone, 1986.

2

Psychiatric Problems in Epilepsy and Their Management

Michael R. Trimble

Epilepsy and psychiatry have always been closely related. The Greeks referred to epilepsy as the sacred disease, because to them only a god could throw a sane, normal man to the ground, deprive him of his senses, convulse him, and then restore him to normality. Hippocrates pointed out that epilepsy was no more sacred than any other disease and ascribed natural causes to it, saying it originated from the brain. In his dissertation on "the sacred disease," he also stated "and men ought to know that from nothing else but thence (from the brain) comes joys, delights, laughter and sports and sorrows, griefs, despondency and lamentations . . . and by the same organ we become mad and delirious and fears and terrors assail us. . . ." He thus firmly placed the origin of both insanity and epilepsy within the brain. In the 19th century, Esquirol, Calmeil, Falret, and Hughlings Jackson established clinical relationships between the two, whereas Kraepelin, in his "Lectures on Clinical Psychiatry," included epileptic insanity as a variety of mental illness. In more recent years, the electroencephalogram was developed initially by a psychiatrist (Hans Berger) and many anticonvulsant drugs used in the treatment of epilepsy have found use in psychiatric patients. These include the barbiturates, phenytoin, valproic acid, carbamazepine, and the benzodiazepines.

The more recent concepts regarding the relationship between epilepsy and psychiatry are summarized in Table 2-1. The late 19th century view, associated with the concept of hereditary degeneration, assumed that patients with epilepsy would automatically show personality change and deterioration. A modern version of this is that only patients with psychomotor seizures, and hence temporal lobe epilepsy, are susceptible to such changes (period of psychomotor peculiarity). This view is contrasted with

Table 2-1. Recent Periods of History Relating Epilepsy
to Psychiatry

Period of epileptic deterioration	−1900
Period of epileptic character	1900–1930
Period of normality	1930–
Period of psychomotor peculiarity	1930–

the position of others who would support the concept that patients with epilepsy are not especially susceptible to developing any psychopathology except that brought about by structural brain damage existing prior to the epilepsy, uncontrolled seizures, prolonged anticonvulsant usage, or the psychosocial stigma of having epilepsy. The period of the epileptic character, namely that which suggested that certain people were constitutionally liable to develop seizures, has now largely passed. This idea was intertwined with some of the more extravagant speculations of psychosomatic medicine, which evolved into a general theory of diseases. Various disease types were specified, such as the peptic ulcer type, the diabetic type, and the epileptic type.

Although in this century the management of chronic epilepsy in some countries has passed from psychiatrists to neurologists, there are four reasons why psychiatrists need to know about epilepsy and its complications. First, the history of the link between epilepsy and psychiatry emphasizes the changing nature of ideas with regard to psychiatric illnesses generally, both as to their supposed pathogenesis and their psychopathological manifestations. Secondly, in any psychiatric setting, patients with epilepsy, particularly chronic epilepsy with continuing uncontrolled seizures, are likely to be seen. Patients in long-stay mental hospitals, patients with mental handicaps in the community, and patients seen by psychiatrists on a liaison service are the most frequent settings for epilepsy to be seen. Thirdly, virtually all of the drugs used in the management of epilepsy, as has been noted, have been used to treat psychopathology, and the anticonvulsant drugs, at least some of them, may also be rightly referred to as psychotropic. Because psychiatrists should have an expertise in medications that affect the mind and behavior, knowledge of anticonvulsants becomes imperative. Finally, some forms of epilepsy, particularly localization-related epilepsy arising from the temporal lobes, are associated with cognitive and behavioral sequelae that closely resemble psychopathology seen in non-epileptic patients.

THE TEMPORAL LOBE STORY

The modern era of epilepsy, and perhaps the most controversial with regard to its relationships to psychiatry, started in the late 1940s with the extensive use of the electroencephalogram, and the reporting by some authors of a high frequency of psychopathology in patients with temporal lobe epilepsy. This, the "period of psychomotor peculiarity," is best summed up by the quotation of Gibbs and Stamps (1953) that "the patient's emotional reactions to his seizures, to his family and his social situation are less important determinants of psychiatric disorder than the site and type of the epileptic discharge."

In contrast, there are authors who have disputed that there is any special relationship between temporal lobe epilepsy and psychopathology, pointing out that, for example, many studies using standardized rating scales such as the Minnesota Multiphasic Personality Inventory (MMPI) for the assessment of psychopathology fail to distinguish between groups of patients with epilepsy. Although there is less disagreement that when, as a group, patients with epilepsy are examined, the prevalence of psychopathology is increased above the normal population, this is attributed to secondary causes outlined above. This debate over the relevance of temporal lobe epilepsy in relationship to psychiatric symptoms has both theoretical and practical implications. Thus, the temporal lobes, particularly the medial temporal structures such as the amygdala and the hippocampus, form part of the limbic system (Fig. 2-1). Around the time

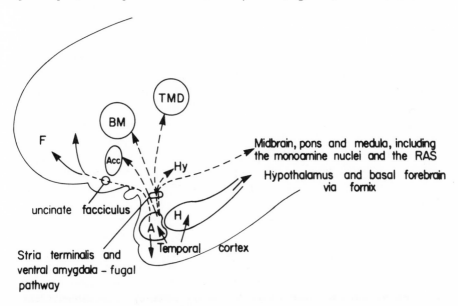

FIG. 2-1. A schematic representation of the amygdala and hippocampus situated medially in the temporal lobe. Some connections are shown, especially to temporal neocortex, the frontal lobes, the limbic forebrain, and the thalamus. A, amygdala; Acc, nucleus accumbens septi; BM, basal nucleus of Meynert; F, frontal and cingulate areas; H, hippocampus; Hy, hypothalamus; TMD, mediodorsal nucleus of the thalamus.

Table 2-2. Components of the
Kluver-Bucy Syndrome

Tameness, loss of fear, and aggression
Hypersexuality
Excessive oral exploration of the environment
Visual agnosia

---

temporal lobe epilepsy was first being investigated with the electroencephalogram, other authors were defining the behavioral consequences of
stimulating or lesioning the temporal lobes. Kluver and Bucy noted their
syndrome, the features of which are shown in Table 2-2, identifying clear-
cut behavior changes which followed pathological destruction of the temporal lobes bilaterally. It was thus reasonable to assume the intactness of
these structures was a prerequisite for the organization and control of
mood, sexual behavior, and visual perception. At the same time, other
animal experiments were outlining the relationship of the amygdala and
hypothalamus to aggression, the hippocampus to memory function, and
neuroanatomists were developing new techniques for tracing and displaying nuclei and related pathways within the brain. The medial temporal
lobe structures were thus seen to be intimately related with forebrain limbic structures, including the so-called "pleasure centers" which, when
stimulated, could provoke continuous self-stimulation by animals to the
point of exhaustion. Thus, alongside the elaboration of the concept of
temporal lobe epilepsy, the idea that the medial temporal lobe structures,
in particular the hippocampus and amygdala which are so often affected
in the pathology of temporal lobe epilepsy, were intimately connected with
behavior and its modulation arose. It was in this climate that the "era of
psychomotor peculiarity" developed, and the idea that it was not all patients with epilepsy who were susceptible to psychiatric illness, but only
those with disturbance of the temporal lobe, in particular limbic system,
structures.

PSYCHIATRIC DISORDERS IN EPILEPSY

The overall spectrum of psychiatric disorders encountered in patients
with epilepsy is essentially no different from the psychiatric disorders encountered in patients without epilepsy. Many of them have clinical characteristics which are typical for traditional psychopathological entities, although there are difficulties with classification. For example, with regard
to *Diagnostic and Statistical Manual of Mental Disorders* classifications (DSM
IIIR), the presence of an underlying brain lesion would automatically ex-
clude the diagnosis of major affective disorder or schizophrenia, and the-

oretically inclusion of these states would have to be under organic mental syndromes. According to the DSM IIIR classifications, however, in that category no specific place is accorded to any particular neurological disease, although there is reason to believe that the psychiatric problems of patients with epilepsy may be special in this regard and may have very close interlinks with psychiatric disorders in the absence of epilepsy.

The most common psychiatric problems encountered in epileptic populations are anxiety, depression, and personality disorders, but the more rare psychoses are of great theoretical interest. Organic mental syndromes, particularly cognitive dulling and dementia are overrepresented in patients with epilepsy. It has become recently appreciated that anticonvulsant drugs themselves may make an important contribution to the development of psychopathology, and this will be highlighted in this chapter. This in itself is not surprising, in the sense that inappropriate use of a number of psychotropic drugs may provoke or increase psychiatric illness. Anticonvulsant drugs traditionally are given for many years, and this brings with it the complications, neurophysiological and metabolic, that arise with the long-term prescription of drugs that affect the central nervous system. Further, the combination of several different compounds, polytherapy, may itself provoke untoward side effects, most notably on cognitive function and mood, in the same way that polytherapy with psychotropic drugs is often counterproductive.

CLASSIFICATION

Psychiatric disorders of epilepsy are best classified in relationship to the seizure itself (Table 2-3). Ictal (peri-ictal) disorders are directly related to the seizure, whereas interictal disorders are unrelated in time to the seizure. A third category would be disorders which, caused by brain disease, lead to both seizures and psychiatric illness. In this latter category are many causes of mental handicap, and some epileptic syndromes such as the Lennox-Gastaut syndrome. This also covers organic mental disorders such as autism and the disintegrative psychosis of childhood, and cerebrovascular disease and Alzheimer's disease in adults.

Ictally Related Disorders

Many of these are manifestations of simple and complex partial seizures in which psychological symptoms predominate. They also include the prodromal symptoms, predominantly affective, and the psychiatric presentations of both generalized absence and complex partial seizure status.

Postictal disorders occur immediately following the seizures when there is usually overt disruption of the EEG, mainly showing diffuse slow frequencies and little normal activity (see Fig. 2-1). Patients present with a

Table 2-3.   Classification of the Psychiatric
Disorders of Epilepsy

Ictal (peri-ictal)
  Prodromata
  Aura
  Postictal
  Partial and generalized absence status
Interictal
  Anxiety-related
  Personality change
  Affective disorders
  Psychoses (bipolar, schizophrenia-like, paranoia)
Secondary to brain disease
  Static
  Progressive

variety of behavior syndromes, the underpinnings of which are related to the detectable confusional states. These are short-lived, but occasionally persist for days or even weeks, and when long-lasting, psychopathology may be seen in the setting of a relatively clear consciousness (see Cases 1 and 2, Chapter 1).

In one study of 100 patients who had ictal emotional experiences, Williams (1956) showed that fear and depression were the most common emotions. The severity of the affective disorder ranged from mild to severe, and in five patients suicidal ideation occurred. Interestingly, ictal depression lasted longer than other ictal epileptic experiences, in several cases going on for longer than 24 hours.

The ictally driven psychoses may be schizophrenia-like, especially in complex partial seizure status, although more often they represent obvious delirium, with a variety of hallucinatory and delusional experiences with evidence of cognitive disorientation in association with the disturbed EEG.

In many patients, transient psychiatric disorders peri-ictally present few problems, although they may be an embarrassment both to the patient and the family. More rarely, such episodes may be prolonged, or so florid as to cause self-damage, and certainly considerable social disadvantages. In such cases, the importance of management is to recognize the relationship of the seizures to the ensuing behavior disorder, and then attempt better seizure control. It is still the case that many patients with chronic epilepsy that come to medical attention have been poorly evaluated with regard to their classification of seizures, their choice of medication, and the amount of the prescription given. It is imperative that such patients be evaluated using the newer techniques of electroencephalographic monitoring and that careful attention be paid to their clinical history.

The two main forms of prolonged EEG monitoring now carried out in the investigation of difficult behavior problems are video telemetry and ambulatory monitoring. In the former, the patient is filmed by a video camera, usually in a specially designed laboratory or ward, and the EEG is simultaneously recorded. Both the picture and the EEG trace are sent to an EEG room where they are displayed on a split screen and viewed together. The EEG and the patient's behavior can thus be correlated.

With ambulatory monitoring, the EEG is recorded for a prolonged period of time using a portable cassette recorder strapped to the patient's body. The technique requires the use of special head-mounted amplifiers that diminish muscle and other artifacts. Although with this method there is no accompanying visual image of the patient, the apparatus can be worn at home or in the school without interference of daily activities. The disadvantage of both of these techniques is the limited number of EEG channels that can be recorded, and the interference that still occurs on the record at crucial times such as during a seizure.

Nonetheless, with such methods it is usually possible to diagnose the patient's seizure type, and to make appropriate prescriptions. Serum-level monitoring may allow subtle but important alterations of anticonvulsant dosage to be made which may bring about the desired reduction of seizure frequency, as may the cautious, but well-thought-out rationalization of unnecessary polypharmacy that the patient may be receiving. It is a common experience that reduction of polypharmacy, rather than leading to an increase in seizures, leads to an overall decrease, with occasional patients being rendered seizure-free by this relatively simple maneuver.

Interictal Psychiatric Disorders

Personality Disorder

As already noted, the views on the relationship between personality change and epilepsy have altered over time, the main arguments revolving around whether the personality changes are part of an organic mental syndrome of epilepsy affecting the temporal lobes, or whether they are caused by secondary factors such as recurrent head injuries, social stigmatization, or the long-term prescription of anticonvulsant drugs. Many studies have been carried out using standardized rating scales such as the MMPI, but few have produced conclusive results. Nonetheless, careful scrutiny of several reportedly negative investigations do show nonsignificant but high levels of psychopathology when a temporal lobe group is compared to a generalized epilepsy group, raised paranoia or schizophrenia scales being quite common. In some studies, psychopathology scores are higher in those with combined psychomotor or generalized seizures or in those with bilateral temporal lobe foci. In general, the data do not support the idea that a specific epileptic personality exists in all patients

Table 2-4.   Components of the
Geschwind Syndrome

Hypergraphia
Hyperreligiosity
Hyposexuality

with temporal lobe epilepsy, but they do suggest that patients with temporal lobe lesions, particularly those with medially sited limbic lesions, are more susceptible to developing severe psychiatric disturbances, among which may be included changes of personality and psychoses.

The view that there is a specific interictal syndrome, particularly of temporal lobe epilepsy, has been most strongly made by Geschwind and colleagues (1979). They included hyposexuality, religiosity, and hypergraphia (a tendency toward extensive and compulsive writing) as common features, noting also a tendency toward philosophical concerns and irritability. Obsessional behavior, circumstantiality, and poor impulse control leading to increased aggressive behavior are also commonly cited (Table 2-4).

Aggression

Historically, paroxysmal disturbances of aggression, in the absence of overt seizures, have often been considered as epileptic equivalents. Impetus for these suggestions has been given by neurosurgical depth electrode studies which show correlations between deep-seated limbic discharges and disturbances of behavior leading to aggression (Fig. 2-2). Thus, the episodic dyscontrol was seen as a consequence of paroxysmal subcortical discharges, not necessarily recorded by the EEG on the surface of the brain. This correlates well with the known anatomical circuits related to aggression in animal studies. These include the medial temporal structures; the evidence from amygdalectomy or anterior temporal lobectomy in man, one of the most common improvements in behavior noted being decreased aggression; and a number of studies showing an increased relationship between aggression and epilepsy, many of which have, however, been criticized on methodological grounds.

Sexual Behavior

The most common sexual disturbance quoted is hyposexuality. Patients with seizures arising from the temporal lobes tend to be more hyposexual than those with major generalized seizures; patients often report a global loss of sexual interest and little concern over this. There are isolated cases of sexual deviation and gender dysphoria being associated with seizures.

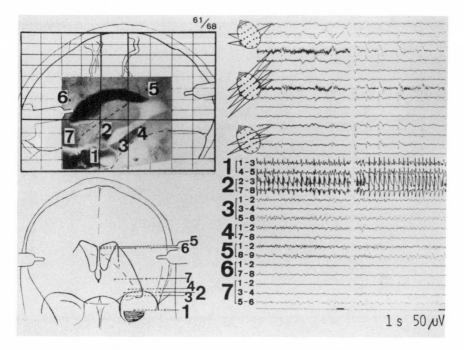

FIG. 2-2. Relationship of aggressive behavior to deep-seated limbic discharges. Placement of electrodes 1 and 2 is in the pre-amygdaloid region of the temporal lobe. Discharges are noted during an aggressive outburst only in this area, not seen on surface electrodes. (Reproduced by permission of H. G. Wieser.)

Any association of hyposexuality with temporal lobe disturbances has to take into account recent findings of low levels of free testosterone in the presence of increased total testosterone and high sex hormone-binding globulin levels in male epileptic patients. The lowest free testosterone levels tend to be seen in patients with "low sex drive," although they are usually within the normal, quoted limits. These findings suggest associations among low libido, temporal lobe dysfunction, and anticonvulsant treatments, particularly in patients with more severe seizure disorders.

Hypergraphia

Of all of the behavior changes described, an increased interest in philosophical matters, a tendency toward religiosity, and hypergraphia are perhaps the most intriguing. Although it is clear that these occur in a minority of patients, their presence may be missed, either on account of the fact that their religious behavior and mystical ruminations are accepted as normal, or their hypergraphia is not carefully sought. Sometimes, patients come to the hospital bearing multiple books with their writings (Figs. 2-3–2-5), often themselves being involved in writing a book that may or

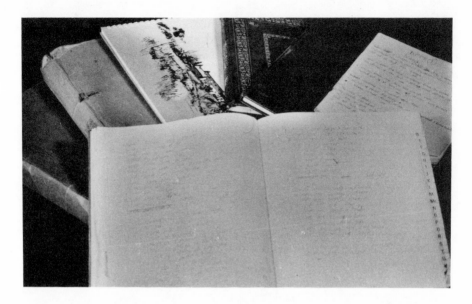

FIG. 2-3. An example of hypergraphia, a tendency toward extensive and compulsive writing.

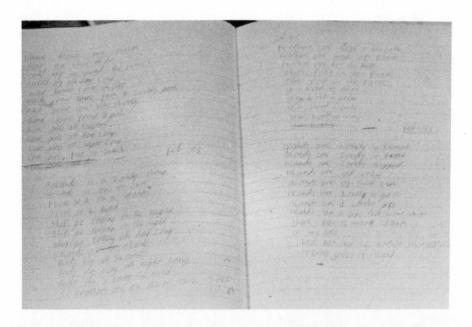

FIG. 2-4. Repetitive and meticulous writing, a common feature of hypergraphia.

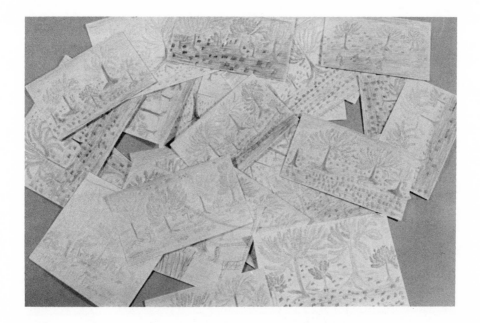

FIG. 2-5. Samples of extensive drawing, a feature of hypergraphia.

may not have some religious theme. The writing is often characteristically meticulous, and may be repetitive. Often patients describe a compulsion to write; however, this may be reflected in alternative ways (e.g., through hiring a public stenographer or through extensive drawing or painting). Studies of the phenomenon are few, but do suggest that it may be associated with a temporal lobe disturbance.

Treatment of patients whose personality change has reached the range of being pathological, and which is disruptive both to themselves and to the society in which they live, can be problematic. Further, as noted, the relative contributions of pathology in the temporal lobes, or continuing disruption of personality development caused by the presence of chronic illness is difficult, in many cases various factors summating. The role of anticonvulsant drugs has to be considered, in particular long-standing prescription of barbiturate-type compounds. There is some experimental evidence that patients receiving carbamazepine are less likely to exhibit the more severely abnormal personality changes, and patients with personality problems and recurrent seizures should, when possible, be treated with monotherapy. Establishing a good rapport with such patients, improving their compliance, and attempting to alter adverse environmental factors are always helpful. Many personality changes (e.g., the religiosity) are not usually a problem and some (e.g., meticulousness) may be socially advantageous, even if recognized as abnormal by the patient's friends and relatives.

Major Affective Disorders

Although some kind of interictal mood change probably represents the most common illness in patients with epilepsy, this is much more frequently dysthymia, rather than major depression. Although no epidemiological study exists of its prevalence, rating scale studies in outpatient settings have revealed a high frequency of depressive symptoms, more so than in patients with other neurological conditions attending the same centers. Trimble and colleagues have recently examined 64 patients with a combined clinical diagnosis of depression and epilepsy seen over a 3-year period to clarify in more detail the phenomenology of the depression, its pathogenesis, and treatment. The severity was regarded as moderate, and it was "endogenous" in approximately 40%. It was associated with high ratings on a hostility rating scale, another important feature being the presence of high anxiety scores. Thirteen patients were psychotic, although bipolar presentations (manic depressives) were rare. This latter finding accords with several other studies which suggest that manic illness in epilepsy is not common, and when it occurs, it is usually associated with a prolonged peri-ictal state, often precipitated by a flurry of epileptic seizures.

It is important to note that the frequency of suicide is increased in epileptic patients, particularly in patients with temporal lobe epilepsy, as is the taking of an overdose. This has some implications for treatment, in the sense that the most common drugs used in overdose are barbiturates, and such abuse may have a fatal outcome.

A number of authors have tried to correlate seizure variables with affective disorder. It has been reported to be more common with late onset epilepsy, and some authors have noted a decline in fit frequency prior to hospitalization for the treatment of major affective disorder. Trimble and colleagues did not report any relationship between the type of seizure, frequency of attacks, and site of lesion and the phenomenology of the depressive illness, although the duration of illness was correlated with severity.

Flor-Henry (1969) suggested a relationship between manic-depressive psychosis and nondominant temporal lobe lesions. When studying patients with temporal lobe epilepsy awaiting surgery, who also had a psychiatric illness, he noted that where lateralization could be determined, 18% were right hemisphere lesions, the majority of whom had a manic-depressive psychosis. Although this has never been replicated, there is some evidence from nonepileptic patients of a link between the nondominant hemisphere and emotional behavior, which lends some support to Flor-Henry's suggestion. However, major depression and dysthymic dis-

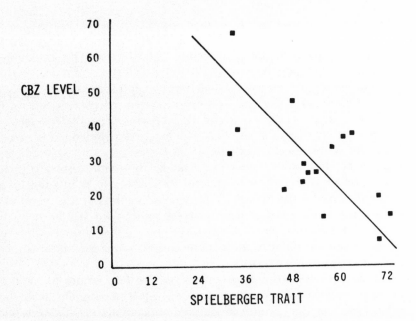

FIG. 2-6. Relationship between carbamazepine serum levels and affective disorder scores on rating scales.

order are probably not associated so clearly with laterality, and in many patients the affective disorder is the outcome of multiple factors. An interesting link relates to folic acid metabolism. It has been long recognized that patients with epilepsy on some anticonvulsant drugs show altered folate metabolism, and several studies have shown a link between psychiatric disturbance and low folate levels in both epileptic and nonepileptic patients. Depressive illness is frequently cited both in children and in adults, not only in institutionalized, but also in outpatient and community studies. To date there is no evidence that folic acid supplements influence the onset or prognosis of the affective state, but S-adenosylmethionine (SAM), a central nervous system (CNS) methyl donor involved in transmethylation reactions which involve folate coenzymes, seems to have antidepressant properties.

Trimble and colleagues noted several relationships between anticonvulsant drugs and mood. Patients receiving phenobarbitone as part of polytherapy were more significantly depressed than those not receiving the drug, whereas patients receiving carbamazepine rated themselves as less depressed and had less guilt. Further, they reported lower trait anxiety scores to patients not receiving carbamazepine. Statistically significant negative correlations between trait anxiety scores and both carbamazepine dose and level were noted (Fig. 2-6).

Several other studies have also noted significant negative correlations between carbamazepine levels and measures of psychopathology. These data are in keeping with the improvement in affective symptoms noted on rationalization of polytherapy, particularly with the removal of barbiturates and the substitution with carbamazepine, and the now known value of carbamazepine in affective disorders in the absence of epilepsy (see Chapter 7). The association between phenobarbitone and depression is also interesting because this has been anecdotally acknowledged for many years but not systematically studied.

In summary, depressive illness, in particular dysthymic disorder, is frequently reported in patients with epilepsy although, except in a few cases, clear identification of the epileptic and neurophysiological underpinnings of this are not clear. One of the strongest associations has been to the prescription of anticonvulsants, although the recurrent seizures which bring continued disappointment to the patient and his persistent social demoralization are contributory factors.

Treatment revolves around three factors. The first relates to rationalization of polytherapy where this is present, and if possible the avoidance of barbiturates and the barbiturate-derived anticonvulsants. There is little excuse these days for prescribing phenobarbitone, and primidone in polytherapy is likely to give the patient a substantial barbiturate serum level. Phenytoin, too, is probably best avoided. Rationalization of the polytherapy, with substitution of the older drugs for carbamazepine, is likely to improve depressive symptoms in many patients.

The second question relates to whether or not antidepressants should be prescribed. In any epilepsy clinic a good proportion of patients will be on antidepressants, but the majority of these lower the seizure threshold and may make the control of epilepsy more difficult. Drugs particularly implicated include maprotiline, mianserin, amitriptyline, clomipramine, and imipramine. Viloxazine appears to have little effect on the seizure threshold but may readily provoke carbamazepine and phenytoin toxicity and is therefore best avoided. In general, if possible, it is best to avoid antidepressants, another good reason being that in patients on hepatic enzyme-inducing anticonvulsants, the serum levels of antidepressant drugs are likely to be low on the usual therapeutic doses.

The third element of treatment relates to increasing the patient's morale with more formal psychotherapy if required. It is often possible, by appropriate therapy and the passage of time, to see the depressive illness resolve without antidepressant drugs. Electroconvulsive therapy (ECT) is not contraindicated and should be used if necessary in patients with major depression, particularly if suicide is a danger. There is a subgroup of patients whose seizure frequency declines markedly before the onset of a severe depressive episode; again, in these, ECTs or the prescription of an epileptogenic drug must be considered.

Anxiety Neurosis and Phobias

As with affective disorders, there are no epidemiological studies that reliably give an estimate of the prevalence of these conditions in epilepsy. Nonetheless, they are frequent and can be very disabling. An important point is that panic attacks can closely resemble a temporal lobe ictal disturbance, where auras of panic and fear are not infrequent. Further, patients with established epilepsy often have panic attacks, which may become confused with simple or complex partial seizures and their escalating frequency may be misinterpreted as a deterioration of the epileptic state.

A biological relationship between anxiety and seizures is suggested in some cases by several lines of evidence. Thus, intracerebral recordings have shown that fear may arise from discharge in limbic brain areas, particularly in the periamygdaloid region. Williams (1956) recorded ictal emotional experiences of 100 patients with epilepsy and noted fear to occur in 61. These emotional experiences were seen mainly with anterior and midtemporal locations of the seizures. The suggestion is that patients with complex or simple partial seizures arising from the temporal lobes may be more susceptible to anxiety and episodes of panic.

Not all anxiety has such associations. In patients with true phobic anxiety related to seizures, an agoraphobia may develop, the patient becoming increasingly housebound and fearful of having attacks in public. There is a small group of patients in whom anxiety precipitates a seizure, and an accelerating cycle of seizures begetting anxiety begetting seizures develops. This can reach the stage of a medical emergency, requiring hospitalization to interrupt the chain of events. The unwary should recognize the multiple manifestations of anxiety, which includes the onset of nonepileptic (pseudo) seizures.

Treatment is initially related to identifying triggers and conflicts and tackling the anxiety directly by behavioral techniques or on occasion with formal psychotherapy. As with depression, studies have shown that rationalization of polytherapy lessens the rating of anxiety symptoms in patients, and an anxiolytic effect of carbamazepine has been shown in several studies (see above). Medications other than anticonvulsants are less helpful, although the benzodiazepine clobazam, which has substantial anticonvulsant as well as anxiolytic properties, may be of value either in the short or the long term.

Psychoses

From the point of view of the psychiatrist, the interictal psychoses are of most interest. Not only do such patients often require active psychiatric treatment, and may thus be presented to psychiatrists with little knowledge of epilepsy as acute medical problems, but also evidence has shown

Table 2-5. Differences Between Process
Schizophrenia and the Schizophrenia-like Psychoses
of Epilepsy

Patients with epilepsy
    Have no evidence of a family history of schizophrenia
    Have no premorbid schizoid personalities
    Maintain their affective responses
    Catatonic phenomena are rare
    Hebephrenic deterioration rare

---

that the interictal psychoses may resemble almost completely the psychoses seen in the absence of epilepsy. They thus become potential biological models for the development of psychosis without epilepsy. Further, depth electrode studies have indicated close associations between epilepsy and psychosis. Psychotic patients without seizures may show abnormal EEGs, including spike wave abnormalities, from subcortical sites in the absence of disturbed cortical rhythms, the onset of the psychosis correlating with spread of the disturbance to specific limbic system sites (e.g., in the limbic forebrain).

Risk factors have been sought by several authors. Hill (1953) and Pond (1975) noted an affinity between temporal lobe epilepsy and a chronic paranoid hallucinatory state and that the epileptic attacks began prior to the onset of the psychosis. Hermann and colleagues (1980) used the MMPI to compare ratings of patients with temporal lobe epilepsy with those with generalized epilepsy, and noted that it was patients with temporal lobe epilepsy and an aura of fear that displayed the most pathological elevations of the rating scale subscores, especially for schizophrenia. Ictal fear is known to be related to activity in medial temporal structures (see above). Other factors suggested from the literature include age of onset of seizures, around or after the age of 10, the presence of automatisms, and sphenoidal, spike wave activity on the electroencephalogram, especially bilateral activity.

The most extensive series reported was that of Slater and colleagues who phenomenologically noted many similarities, and also some differences, between the schizophrenia-like psychosis of epilepsy and process schizophrenia. Thus, the former had an absence of abnormal premorbid schizoid personality traits or a family history of psychiatric disturbance that might suggest a predisposition to schizophrenia, and catatonic phenomena were rare although affective responses were warm and preserved (Table 2-5). However, the majority of their series had a psychosis that was highly typical of paranoid schizophrenia, and some associations to epilepsy variables were noted. The mean age of onset of the psychosis was

Table 2-6. The First-Rank Symptoms of Schneider

The hearing of one's thoughts spoken aloud in one's head
The hearing of voices commenting on what one is doing at the time
Voices arguing in the third person
Experiences of bodily influence
Thought withdrawal and other forms of thought interference
Thought diffusion
Delusional perception[a]
Everything in the spheres of feeling, drive, and volition that the patient experiences is imposed on him or influenced by others

---

[a]An abnormal significance attached to a real perception without any cause that is understandable in rational or emotional terms.

29.8 years, and it occurred after the epilepsy had been present for a mean of 14.1 years. Other authors have also noted that the psychosis usually occurs after the onset of the epilepsy. In some 25% of cases, the psychotic symptoms appeared when the frequency of the generalized seizures were falling. No associations to anticonvulsant prescriptions were noted. The majority of their cases had some disturbance of temporal lobe function and a diagnosis of temporal lobe epilepsy.

The phenomenology of these disorders has been examined in much more detail by Trimble and colleagues (1980). In a prospective study of epileptic psychoses, occurring in the presence of clear consciousness and lasting for at least a month, using a semistandardized rating scale, it has been shown that some 50% of patients will have a typical schizophrenia-like illness, 92% having a profile of nuclear schizophrenia based on the first-rank symptoms of Schneider. The latter are recognized criteria used for the diagnosis of schizophrenia mainly in Anglo-Saxon countries, which represent disorders of thought, specific delusions, and certain auditory hallucinations (Table 2-6). This group also recognized the preservation of affective responses, generally confirming the findings of Slater and Beard (1963). Patients with the nuclear syndrome were more likely to be living at home, or be at work, and were less inclined to show intellectual deterioration than patients with other forms of psychoses.

Flor-Henry suggested that patients with epilepsy and temporal lobe lesions who were psychotic were more likely to be schizophreniform if they had a left-sided lesion. Interestingly, this laterality finding has been substantiated by several authors. Its importance rests in the relevance of the dominant hemisphere for understanding the development of psychosis in patients who do not have epilepsy, and in confirming the biological nature of the link between psychosis and epilepsy in epileptic patients. In other words, the laterality findings are not well explained in terms of sociological concepts of psychiatric illness, and more likely suggest biological links between the psychosis and the epilepsy.

The issue then becomes as to whether both (psychosis and epilepsy) are the outcome of some underlying lesion, or whether the epilepsy itself leads on to the development of psychosis. The former point of view has been supported by several authors including Slater and Beard (1963), mainly on the grounds that patients with the psychosis are more likely to demonstrate a clearly defined organic lesion, often in the temporal lobe. Thus, the psychotic symptoms, and the epileptic seizures, both become epiphenomena of the same or a similar or a related pathological process. The siting of the lesion is crucial, implicating the temporal lobe-limbic system. The alternative hypothesis has been supported by others including Flor-Henry. Evidence for it includes the inverse relationship between the frequency of seizures and the onset of psychosis seen in some patients; the depth electrode studies, which reveal abnormal electrical activity in deep temporal lobe structures in association with psychotic behavior, and the obvious fact that in psychiatry a seizure, albeit artificially induced, is used to resolve a psychosis in patients with severe affective disorder. Further, recent studies using both positron emission tomography and magnetic resonance imaging (MRI) in patients with epilepsy and psychosis have revealed the following. Interictal hypometabolic areas are seen in patients with temporal lobe epilepsy and are quite extensive. They involve several limbic system-related areas from temporal cortex to frontal cortex and the basal ganglia on the side of the focus. Psychotic patients tend to show lower values for the regional cerebral blood flow and regional metabolic rate of oxygen utilization on the left side in the temporal cortex, a finding not seen in nonpsychotic control groups. MRI scans show there is little difference in any brain areas of quantitated T1 values (one measure derived from these scans) between patients with and without psychosis, implying that gross structural lesions do not identify the psychotic group.

Summarizing, it is clear that a small group of patients develop epileptic psychoses, and in some of these the terms schizophrenia-like is appropriate. It is most likely to be related to seizure factors, in particular a site of origin of seizures in the temporal lobe, their spread, their expression as complex partial seizures, and interictal disturbances within limbic system structures outside the immediate temporal lobe areas.

Treatment relates very much to the type of psychosis present and the relationship to the ictus. Clearly, peri-ictal psychoses require better control of the seizures to prevent recurrence. The temporary institution of an antipsychotic drug such as haloperidol may be of value to control behavior, and attempts to improve patient compliance if this is seen to be problematic are imperative. The interictal psychoses are treated as are psychiatric disorders in the absence of epilepsy with a few singular exceptions. Manic-depressive psychoses (which are rare) may be treated with lithium, although rationalization of polytherapy and the introduction of carbamazepine would appear to be logical. Paranoid and schizophrenia-like psychoses should be evaluated from the point of view of the relationship to seizure frequency. Patients who stop having seizures or who have a diminished seizure frequency prior to the onset of the psychosis require a neuroleptic medication which lowers the seizure threshold, namely a phenothiazine such as chlorpromazine. Such patients occasionally require the application of ECT, particularly if their psychosis is life-threatening. Alternatively, patients who have an increase, or no alteration of their seizure frequency in association with interictal psychoses require a neuroleptic drug less likely to precipitate seizures. Generally, these are the butyrophenones including haloperidol and pimozide. The substituted benzamide, sulpiride, is also of value. Longer acting intramuscular preparations such as flupentixol decanoate can be used, and to date, there is no evidence that they interfere with the control of seizures or upset serum anticonvulsant levels.

ALCOHOL WITHDRAWAL SEIZURES

It is commonly acknowledged that withdrawal of alcohol, particularly in people who have abused it, may lead to seizures. This is but one of the relationships between alcohol and seizures, but it emphasizes the importance of using medications during the withdrawal phase that have anticonvulsant as opposed to convulsant properties. In the study of Victor and Brausch (1967) (see Fig. 2-7), almost 50% of the patients had seizures occurring between 13 and 24 hours after cessation of the drinking, the majority of the attacks occurring in under 36 hours. However, in some cases the seizures may be delayed for a matter of days. They usually occur after a period of comparative or absolute abstinence, and the seizure is most often of a generalized nature. In cases of delirium tremens, seizures often occur prior to the delirium. The EEG is usually abnormal, showing oversensitivity to photic stimulation.

Alternative relationships between alcohol and seizures should also be considered, e.g., seizures occurring in established epilepsy following excessive drinking, or the development of seizures in the posttraumatic setting following head injury secondary to alcohol intoxication. Victor and Brausch (1967) proposed that alcoholic epilepsy was a separate entity, secondary to alcohol-related brain damage. Clinical studies of alcoholics with seizures find that alcohol withdrawal only accounts for a percentage of seizures, and some patients, with no apparent predisposition to epilepsy, have a seizure disorder unrelated to withdrawal. Some authors refer to this as alcoholic epilepsy.

In the withdrawal setting, medications with anticonvulsant properties are recommended to prevent the occurrence of seizures. In addition to

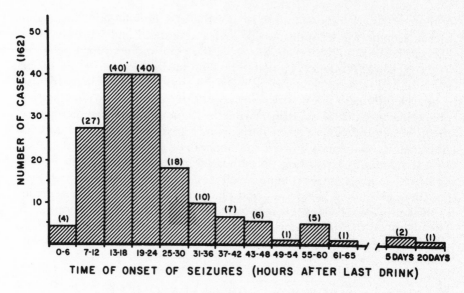

FIG. 2-7. Time of onset of seizures after cessation of drinking is shown. (Reproduced with permission from Victor and Brausch, 1967.)

the seizures, however, treatment should also be aimed at minimizing subjective withdrawal symptoms, and preventing other complications such as cardiac arrhythmias and psychosis. A list of drugs used includes barbiturates, paraldehyde, phenothiazines, butyrophenones, benzodiazepines, and anticonvulsants. The benzodiazepines, including the anticonvulsant benzodiazepines diazepam, lorazepam, and clobazam, are relatively safe and have cross-tolerance with alcohol. Their anticonvulsant protection is of value, but the recent descriptions of dependence related to benzodiazepines makes them less viable alternatives in the treatment of patients with a known dependency syndrome. Both phenytoin and carbamazepine have also been used, and in some countries carbamazepine is the drug most widely prescribed as an anticonvulsant in the withdrawal phase. In addition to effectively controlling seizures, there is no cross-tolerance to alcohol and carbamazepine has no dependence-inducing properties. Further, it decreases the target withdrawal symptoms that occur with alcoholism, perhaps reflective of some psychotropic effect.

The main aim of treatment is to reach a therapeutic serum level as soon as possible, and to maintain seizure protection for a sufficient period of time. If carbamazepine syrup is used initially, protection is achieved within 2 hours, following which the anticonvulsant can be administered in tablet form in doses of 800–1,200 mg. Following the alcohol withdrawal period, the medication may be slowly tapered off, although if the alcohol abuse is interlinked with mood instability, long-term maintenance on carbamazepine may be of value. In patients with identified alcoholic epilepsy, carbamazepine monotherapy would seem to be a logical prescription.

ANTICONVULSANT DRUGS, COGNITIVE FUNCTION, AND ENCEPHALOPATHY

It has become clear recently that, although many patients with epilepsy retain normal intellectual functions, a number show selective areas of cognitive deficit, or a more insidious generalized decline. There has also been substantial literature emphasizing that many anticonvulsant drugs can impair cognitive functions, not only in patients but also in healthy volunteers. The selective cognitive domains that have been examined are those of memory, attention, perceptuomotor skills, and arithmetical and reading attainment skills, the latter mainly in children. Speed of mental processing, although not a distinct domain of abilities, is often of crucial importance in the execution of psychological tests, and there are many references in the literature to people with epilepsy showing "slowness of mental reaction," sometimes referred to as stickiness of thought or mental viscosity. This forms a central component of subcortical dementia, a condition which is more and more becoming recognized as important in a number of neuropsychiatric conditions, and affects a small number of people with epilepsy.

The precise nature of the memory disturbances in epilepsy is difficult to clarify, but patients usually complain of difficulty in recalling recently learned events, and forgetfulness for everyday things. There is some evidence suggesting that memory deficits are more common following temporal lobe lesions, and certainly following temporal lobectomy, selected deficits of memory functions can be detected.

Impairments of attention, in the absence of overt seizures, have been frequently described and are important to recognize in epileptic children with poor educational attainment. Such attentional problems have been described more in patients with generalized seizures than with focal seizures, although not all studies have replicated this observation. Recognition of poor arithmetical ability, or reading attainment below that expected for the child's age and educational standards are important therapeutically, and should always be assessed in new patients.

The majority of patients with epilepsy are maintained on anticonvulsant drugs for many years, and it is now known that this in itself may affect cognitive function, although in a rather nonspecific way. Thus, patients on polytherapy tend to show more impairments of performance, across a wide spectrum of testing abilities, than people on monotherapy. Demonstrable improvements in cognitive function may be shown following rationalization of polytherapy, particularly when carbamazepine is substituted for one or all of the existing anticonvulsant drugs that a patient is

Table 2-7.   Improvement on Some Cognitive Tasks When Patients on Polytherapy Had Carbamazepine Substituted for One or Two of Their Drugs

Significant changes in test scores between the three sessions for the drug reduction patients	
Psychological tests for attention and memory	
Attention (visual scanning)	
Alone	1v3;2v3[a]
With auditory task	1v3;2v3[a]
Total number scanned	1v3[a]
Total number of errors	1v3[a]
Memory (pictures)	
Delayed recall	1v3[a]
Psychological tests for mental and motor speed	
Mental speed	
Perceptual speed for words	1v2;1v3[b]
Decision making for color	1v3[a]
Decision making for category	1v3[a]
Motor speed (tapping rate)	
Dominant hand	1v2;1v3[c]
Nondominant hand	1v2;1v3[b]
Both hands	1v2;1v3[b]

1 = base-line session. 2 = 3 months after drug substitution.
3 = 6 months after substitution.
[a] $p < 0.05$. [b] $p < 0.01$. [c] $p < 0.001$.

receiving. In the investigations of Trimble and Bolwig (1986), the substitution of carbamazepine in patients on polytherapy led to a significant improvement in a number of cognitive tasks (Table 2-7). Such changes tend to be long-term, and not acute, and may be associated with an improvement of seizure frequency.

In investigations of the drug-induced changes of cognitive function in nonepileptic volunteers, and in patients shown in Fig. 1-4, there are differences between anticonvulsant drugs. Carbamazepine has the least number of effects, maximum problems being shown with phenytoin.

Findings such as these suggest that certain patients, especially on drugs like phenytoin, may function better with neuropsychological testing when changed to carbamazepine, and if they are to receive drugs like phenobarbitone or phenytoin, serum levels should be kept to a minimum. These results also suggest carbamazepine may have a different pattern of effect on neuropsychological tests than some of the other drugs. Thus, there is a suggestion that phenytoin, and valproic acid at higher serum levels, leads to a general slowing of cognitive processes, which if severe enough, would

Table 2-8. Relationships Among Anticonvulsant Drugs, Behavior, and Cognitive Function

Drugs	Cognitive function	Behavior
Carbamazepine	Minimal effects	Psychotropic
Clobazam	Minimal effects	Psychotropic
Clonazepam	Impairs	Hyperactivity, conduct disturbance
Ethosuximide	Variable	May provoke psychosis
Phenobarbitone	Impairs	Affective disorder, hyperactivity
Phenytoin	Impairs	Affective disorder
Valproic acid	Minimal effects	Psychotropic (?)

interfere with performance on daily activities. Carbamazepine has fewer widespread effects, and these do not appear to relate to mental speed. The fact that many patients with epilepsy show slowing of their ability to perform cognitive tasks is clearly important, since any drug effect for this should be minimized.

An associated, but much rarer problem, is that of an insidious encephalopathy which may develop in some patients with severe epilepsy. This is probably more common in those with mental retardation and patients with intractable seizures receiving polypharmacy for many years. The cognitive decline is such that the term, dementia, would be appropriate for some cases, although the deterioration is often arrested. The importance of recognizing the syndrome is that it is partially reversible by removing the offending anticonvulsant drugs (phenytoin being the most implicated), the term, dilantin dementia, being introduced for this state at one time.

In summary, anticonvulsant drugs may have deleterious effects on cognitive functions in patients with epilepsy, although this is more related to some drugs than others. This should be viewed as separate but related to their influence on behavior. For example, their propensity both to improve behavior in patients with affective disorder (e.g., carbamazepine), and to lead to a deterioration of behavior (e.g., the provocation of an affective disorder in adults or conduct disturbance in children by phenobarbitone). Some of these relationships are summed up in Table 2-8.

REFERENCES AND SUGGESTED READING

Barraclough B. Suicide and epilepsy. In: Reynolds EH, Trimble MR, eds. *Epilepsy and Psychiatry*. Edinburgh: Churchill Livingstone, 1981:72–76.

Blumer D, Walker AE. The neural basis of sexual behaviour. In: Benson DF, Blumer D, eds. *Psychiatric Aspects of Neurologic Disease*. Orlando, FL: Grune & Stratton, 1975:199–217.

Edeh J, Toone BK. Antiepileptic therapy, folate deficiency and psychiatric morbidity: a general practice survey. *Epilepsia* 1985;26:434–440.

Flor-Henry P. Psychosis and temporal lobe epilepsy: a controlled investigation. *Epilepsia* 1969;10:363–395.

Gallhofer B, Trimble MR, Frackowiak R, Gibbs J, Jones T. A study of cerebral blood flow and metabolism in epileptic psychosis using positron emission tomography and oxygen. *J Neurol Neurosurg Psychiatry* 1985;48:201–206.

Geschwind N. Behavioural changes in temporal lobe epilepsy. *Psychol Med* 1979;9:217–219.

Gibbs FA, Stamps FW. *Epilepsy Handbook.* Springfield, IL: Charles C Thomas, 1953.

Guerrant J, Anderson J, Fischer A, Weinstein MR, Jaros RM, Deskins A. *Personality in Epilepsy.* Springfield, IL: Charles C Thomas, 1962.

Heath RG. Psychosis and epilepsy: similarities and differences in the anatomic-physiologic substrate. In: Koella WP, Trimble MR, eds. *Temporal Lobe Epilepsy, Mania and Schizophrenia and The Limbic System.* Basel: Karger, 1982:106–116.

Hermann B, Schwartz MS, Karnes WE, et al. Psychopathology in epilepsy: relationship of seizure type to age of onset. *Epilepsia* 1980;21:15–23.

Hill D. Psychiatric disorders of epilepsy. *Med Press* 1953;229:473–475.

Perez MM, Trimble MR. Epileptic psychosis-diagnostic comparison with process schizophrenia. *Br J Psychiatry* 1980;137:245–249.

Perez MM, Trimble MR, Reider I, Murray NM. Epileptic psychosis, a further evaluation of PSE profiles. *Br J Psychiatry* 1984;146:155–163.

Pond DA; Psychiatric aspects of epilepsy. *J Indian Med Assoc* 1975;3:1441–1451.

Reynolds EH, Trimble MR. *Epilepsy and Psychiatry.* Edinburgh: Churchill Livingstone, 1981.

Robertson MM, Trimble MR, Townsend HRA. The phenomenology of depression in epilepsy. *Epilepsia* 1987;28:264–272.

Slater E, Beard AW. The schizophrenia-like psychoses of epilepsy. *Br J Psychiatry* 1963;109:95–150.

Tempkin O. *The Falling Sickness.* Baltimore: Johns Hopkins Press, 1971.

Trimble MR. Non-MAOI antidepressants in epilepsy. *Epilepsia* 1978;19:241–250.

Trimble MR. *Biological Psychiatry.* Chichester: John Wiley & Sons, 1988.

Trimble MR, Bolwig TG. *Aspects of Epilepsy and Psychiatry.* Chichester: John Wiley & Sons, 1986.

Trimble MR, Corbett JA, Donaldson J. Folic acid and mental symptoms in children with epilepsy. *J Neurol Neurosurg Psychiatry* 1980;43:1030–1034.

Trimble MR, Perez MM. Psychosocial functioning in adults. In: Kulig B et al., eds. *Epilepsy and Behaviour.* Amsterdam: Swets & Zeitlinger, 1980:118–126.

Victor M, Brausch C. The role of abstinence in the genesis of alcohol epilepsy. *Epilepsia* 1967;8:1–20.

Williams D. The structure of emotions reflected in epileptic experiences. *Brain* 1956;79:29–67.

3

Principles of Applied Clinical Pharmacology: A Guide to Therapeutics

C. E. Pippenger

Clinicians have had a long-standing interest in establishing why a fixed drug dosage is therapeutically effective in some individuals but not in others. For years, appropriate dosage regimens of drugs were established only by the empirical trial and error approach. Modern analytical techniques provide an alternative to empirical drug therapy. Our ability to correlate serum or plasma drug concentrations (and by inference tissue concentrations) with the observed clinical effect of a given agent has provided new insights into all aspects of therapeutics. Historically, the measurement of serum drug concentrations was one of the functions of the clinical pharmacology research laboratory, but the increasing demand for such measurements to be performed routinely has exceeded the capacity of these laboratories. Over the last decade, the demand for this procedure has increased geometrically to the point where therapeutic drug monitoring has evolved into a routine diagnostic test. Today, special sections within most hospital clinical chemistry laboratories are available to provide routine drug-monitoring services.

Utilizing the new drug-monitoring techniques, we have a better understanding of the interrelationships between the drug dose and its pharmacological effect. For many drugs, the desired therapeutic (pharmacological) effect is achieved only after a specific plasma concentration range for successful drug therapy. Above this range, patients may begin to experience undesirable drug side effects. Below this range, patients may fail to achieve the desired relief from the disease or symptom for which they are receiving therapy. Rapid advances in clinical pharmacology over the past decade are directly attributable to therapeutic drug monitoring (TDM); the clinical efficacy of TDM, in turn, is directly related to the continued rapid advancement in technology associated with the quantitation of drug compounds.

Not until the late 1960s did TDM become widespread. Gas-liquid chromatography (GLC) represented the first major breakthrough because it provided a method of rapidly separating and quantitating individual drugs within a given class. Gas-liquid chromatographic techniques were further refined and improved so that by the early 1970s, GLC analysis of various therapeutically monitored agents was performed routinely in many hospital laboratories. The major disadvantage of GLC was the complexity of the instrumentation, which necessitated a highly trained and skilled analyst. More recent advances in the development of the nitrogen-phosphorus detector, megabore and capillary columns, automatic injectors, and data reduction systems have increased the operational efficiency and sensitivity of the instruments to such an extent that drug analyses can be performed routinely on microvolumes of plasma. However, GLC today is considered primarily a research technique.

The development of radioimmunoassay techniques also permitted quantitation of drug concentrations in microvolumes of serum. Unfortunately, the complexity of the technique, the safety and regulatory problems associated with the use of radioactivity, as well as lack of radioimmunoassays for a wide variety of drugs have prevented its widespread adaptation for routine drug monitoring.

Making TDM available to all laboratories and physicians required simple technology that could be performed by a technician without special training or instrumentation. This was achieved with the development by the Syva Company of the homogeneous enzyme immunoassay technique (EMIT®), which is capable of performing quantitative drug assays on less than $40\mu l$ of serum. The major advantages of the system are its microcapability, accuracy, and the rapidity and ease of operation of the assays. More recently, other immunoassays including substrate-labeled fluorescent immunoassays (SLFIA) (Ames Co.) and fluorescence polarization immunoassays (FPI) (Abbott Diagnostics), which are commonly called TDX assays for the rapid quantitation of drugs, have become available.

A large number of drugs exist for which antibodies are not available, but that must be therapeutically monitored. The most promising and practical method of monitoring these agents is by high-performance (pressure) liquid chromatography (HPLC). Within the last 15 years, the development of HPLC has provided laboratories with a system having the same advantages as the homogeneous enzyme immunoassay systems: it is capable of processing microsamples ($100\mu l$), it is rapid and specific, and the instrumentation is relatively simple to operate as well as being cost-effective. In addition, HPLC can be adapted to simultaneously quantitate a large variety of drugs as well as their active and inactive metabolites. It is a valuable tool for establishing correlations between drug and drug metabolite concentrations in biological fluids.

Table 3-1.   Indications for Monitoring Plasma Drug Levels

Plasma drug levels should be monitored for the following reasons:
  When a drug has a narrow, well-defined therapeutic range
  When noncompliance is suspected
  When the desired therapeutic effect is not achieved or when symptoms of toxicity
    are observed
  When there are large interindividual variations in drug utilization or metabolism
  When a drug utilization is altered as a consequence of secondary disease or
    changing physiological state
  When drug interaction is suspected
  When there is a need for medicolegal verification of treatment
  When plasma concentrations associated with optimal response need to be defined

---

As with any new laboratory discipline, TDM is not a panacea that will solve all problems associated with drug therapy. There are specific clinical applications just as there are situations where it will probably serve no useful purpose. TDM is most applicable when the drug in question has a narrow therapeutic range, is used chronically, has potentially toxic side effects if overdosed, and has minimal therapeutic effects if underdosed. The clinical indications for monitoring a patient's drug concentrations are summarized in Table 3-1. Both clinical and molecular studies of the pharmacological profiles of a wide variety of drugs have demonstrated that a much better correlation exists between the observed clinical effects of a drug and its plasma concentration than that observed between the clinical effect and total daily drug dosage. With this in mind, therapeutic drug monitoring can be utilized to:

Allow the clinician to appropriately compensate for individual variations in drug utilization patterns. If the plasma concentrations following a specific dosage are analyzed in a large patient population, the distribution of drug levels at steady state will be gaussian. The vast majority of patients will have levels within the range expected from that dosage based on their body weight (mg/kg). Patients who are genetically either "fast" or "slow" drug metabolizers will have levels at the extreme ends of the curve. Fast drug metabolizers require higher doses to achieve the same plasma concentrations and consequently the desired therapeutic effect. Slow drug metabolizers become intoxicated and experience adverse side effects from standard therapeutic doses of the drugs and, therefore, can be maintained at optimal drug levels on dosages well below the standard regimen.

Allow the clinicians to compensate for altered drug utilization associated with various disease states. Patients on long-term drug therapy become acutely ill and are prescribed additional therapeutic agents to control the acute illness. Drug interactions between the acutely and chronically administered drugs may then cause these patients to respond in an unexpected manner to a fixed dosage of medication. The given disease may affect dramatically the drug utilization pattern of any drug, thus altering the pharmacological effect. Acute or chronic uremia dramatically decreases the elimination of drugs that are primarily dependent on urinary excretion, and renal failure alters the binding of many drugs to albumin. In both situations, the ratio of free drug to total drug may increase to the point where free drug concentrations are high enough to produce a clinically evident drug response, although the total serum drug concentrations are below the accepted optimal therapeutic range. Moreover, free drug levels can rise into the toxic range to precipitate adverse side effects even though the total drug concentrations remain within or even below the usual ranges.

Hepatic disease can extensively alter a given therapeutic response by impairing a patient's ability to metabolize drugs. Most drugs depend on liver detoxification for conversion to water-soluble products, which are easily eliminated from the body. Thus, a precipitous rise in parent drug concentrations can occur as the drug, which normally would have been metabolized by the liver and then eliminated from the system, accumulates.

Allow the clinician to adjust therapeutic drug regimens to compensate for changing physiological states. Normal alterations in physiological state also change drug utilization patterns. TDM is crucial to successful dosage adjustment of therapeutic regimens in pregnancy, neonates, children, and the elderly.

Recent studies have shown that decreased drug absorption during pregnancy is associated with a decrease in serum phenytoin concentration and an exacerbation of seizures in epileptic gravidas. The use of TDM from the onset of pregnancy, with appropriate dosage regulation to maintain therapeutic drug concentrations, significantly decreases the number of seizures that occur, thus decreasing potential harm to the fetus.

The normal process of maturation involves a large number of physiological changes that can dramatically alter drug utilization. Complex changes in drug utilization patterns occur in the weeks following birth. Infants and children utilize drugs at a faster rate than adults, and therefore dependent upon age, require from 2 to 10 times as much drug on a body weight (mg/kg) basis as an adult to achieve the same therapeutic drug concentration. As a child enters puberty, drug utilization patterns rapidly change. By early pubescence (between Tanner stages 0 and 1) the conversion to adult drug metabolism patterns is usually complete. These changes usually occur between the ages of 10 and 13, appearing earlier in girls than in boys. We emphasize that although children in the early pubertal stages physically look like children, their physiological status with respect to drug metabolism is that of an adult. Even though it takes years to develop the full secondary sex characteristics associated with maturation, the conversion to adult drug metabolism patterns occurs within a few months (between Tanner 0 and 1). Chronic medication must be administered carefully, with frequent blood level determinations, when treating early pubescent children. Failure to adjust the child's therapeutic regimen to compensate for the associated physiological changes may result in exposure to unnecessary and prolonged drug toxicity, with its attendant sequelae.

As the maturation process continues and the efficiency of normal physiological functions decrease, so does the body's ability to clear drugs efficiently to bind drugs to plasma protein. Geriatric patients often exhibit reduced rates of hepatic drug metabolism and renal drug elimination, thereby requiring reduced drug dosages. The geriatric patient's ability to bind drugs to plasma proteins decreases; therefore, the aged may have total drug plasma concentrations within the optimal therapeutic range, but elevated free drug concentrations that can produce adverse side effects. The clinical signs of drug intoxication in the elderly often present clinically as lethargy and confusion, and TDM provides a means of distinguishing drug-induced confusion from organic deterioration.

It is to be emphasized that although the rate of drug disposition in children is increased, the optimal serum drug concentration of most therapeutic agents necessary to produce the desired therapeutic response is similar to that observed in adults. Therefore, because of the faster drug clearance in children, it is necessary to prescribe larger drug doses (mg/kg) to the pediatric population in order to achieve and maintain optimal drug concentrations, whereas in geriatric patients, lower drug doses are usually necessary to avoid drug toxicity.

Allow the clinician to recognize noncompliance. Many patients, in particular those who have chronic disease which requires consistent drug therapy over a prolonged period of time, tend not to take their medications as prescribed. Moreover, patients with a chronic disease that does not chronically cause pain or other unusual discomfort (e.g., the epilepsies, asthma, hypertension, or mental illness) may easily neglect to take their medicine. The end result of such noncompliance is an exacerbation of the existing disorder at some time in the future. Studies have clearly demonstrated that noncompliance is a major factor in treatment failures. It is well recognized that 60–70% of patients do not take their medications as prescribed by their physician.

Allow the clinician to identify the base-line drug concentrations associated with an optimal therapeutic regimen. After a patient has had an appropriate therapeutic regimen defined, the physician can establish the base-line drug concentration at which the patient achieves the desired therapeutic effect. Should the patient return in the future with the same condition uncontrolled, the physician can rapidly document whether the patient has been compliant, or whether a new disease state has altered the pharmacological response to the drug.

Numerous factors, including individual differences in drug metabolism and excretion, age, sex, patient compliance, disease, and drug interactions (particularly during multiple drug therapy) regulate the drug's disposition pattern within each individual patient. The rate of drug disposition in turn regulates the plasma and tissue concentration and thus, the amount of drug available to interact with specific receptors. The therapeutic response observed in a given patient is dependent on the sum of all these processes, and is directly related to the drug concentration in that particular patient. Interactions among all the potential factors influencing drug disposition account for the broad interpatient variability in plasma concentrations following either single or multiple drug doses. Individual patient response to a given drug dose, however, remains constant because the factors that can alter drug utilization within each individual are relatively fixed.

Generally, interindividual variations of response, as demonstrated by the clinical response of a large population to a fixed drug dose, are a reflection of the relationship between total daily dose and plasma concentrations more than they are of the relationship between plasma concentration and the intensity of the pharmacological response. In other words, the probability of achieving a given plasma concentration from a given drug dose is much less than the probability of obtaining a specific biological effect from a given plasma concentration. This is why there are marked variations in the observed therapeutic response within a population when an average or standard drug dosage is administered to a large number of patients. The desired therapeutic effect will be achieved in some patients; no therapeutic effect will occur in others, because drug clearance is rapid and therapeutic plasma concentrations are never achieved. Conversely, others will show marked drug side effects which are attributable to elevated plasma concentrations because the patient's drug clearance is slow.

PHARMACODYNAMICS: SITE AND MECHANISMS OF DRUG ACTION

The biological effect achieved following a given drug dose is a direct consequence of the formation of reversible bonds between the drug and tissue receptors controlling a particular response. For most drugs, the intensity and duration of a given pharmacological effect is proportional to the drug concentration at the receptor site. The exact mechanism of receptor interactions, however, remains unclear. In order for a drug to exert the desired therapeutic effect, it must reach and interact with the receptors regulating that specific response. In addition, disease, age, sex, compliance, drug interactions, and individual differences in drug metabolism and excretion contribute to interpatient response differences. Figure 3-1 schematically depicts the factors that can alter the concentration of drugs ultimately achieved and maintained at a given receptor site. The titration of drug dosage using plama concentrations thus indirectly influ-

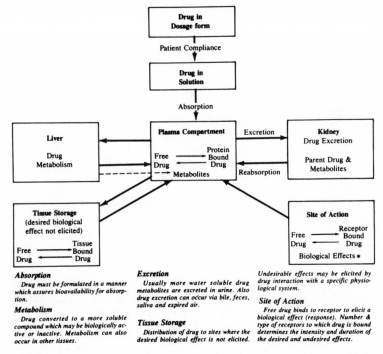

FIG. 3-1. Scheme depicting the factors that can alter the concentrations of drugs ultimately achieved and maintained at a given receptor site.

ences the concentration at receptor sites (see below) and thus reduces interindividual variations in response.

Every drug acts to produce a change in some known physiological function or process. Any drug may increase, decrease, or return to normal the physiological function of tissues, organs, or physiological systems. The biological effect observed following administration of a drug is the sum of the processes by which that drug creates changes in some physiological or biochemical process. Such effects can only be measured and expressed in terms of alteration of a specific function or process. A change in function caused by a drug's pharmacodynamic activity may return the function or physiological process from abnormal to a normal level of activity. Or, it may prevent deviation from the normal physiological state of a given system. For most drugs, the intensity of a pharmacological effect tends to be proportional to the drug concentration present in extracellular fluid which is available to enter tissues and interact with specific receptors to elicit a biological effect. For example, antiepileptic drugs are believed to prevent seizures by binding to neural membranes and/or altering neurotransmitter release. Alteration of these functions is thought to prevent or reduce the spread of the excessive electrical activity that is responsible for precipitating a clinical seizure.

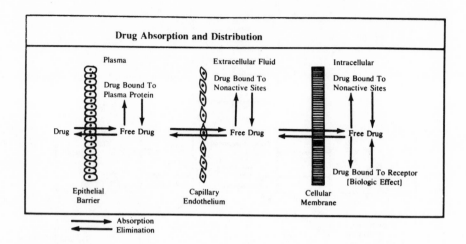

FIG. 3-2. Drug distribution between plasma and tissue.

Following absorption, a drug distributes between the plasma and various tissue compartments (Fig. 3-2). Because many drugs are partially bound to plasma proteins, an equilibrium exists between the concentration of protein-bound drug and the free drug concentration in plasma water. The drug concentration in plasma water is in equilibrium with the drug concentration in extracellular water. Only a free drug is capable of crossing the various lipoprotein membranes that surround the receptor sites. It is impossible to directly monitor receptor-site drug concentrations *in vivo*, but total plasma drug concentrations reflect the equilibrium that exists among tissue, extracellular fluid, and plasma-water-drug concentrations, whereas plasma-free drug levels actually represent the plasma-water-drug concentration and thus reflect levels in the extracellular space. Measuring the free drug concentration is thus an indirect measure of drug concentration at the *site of action,* which may be defined as the site at which a given drug acts to initiate the events that lead to a specific biological effect. A drug's biological effect may be elicited by direct interaction with a receptor that controls a specific function, or by alteration of the physiological process that regulates that specific function.

The *mechanism of action* of a drug refers to the actual biochemical or physical process that initiates a biological response at a specific site. The mechanism of action of most drugs depends upon their chemical interaction with a functionally viable component of some physiological system. However, because the exact molecular mechanism by which drugs interact with receptors remains obscure, theoretical models have been developed to explain their mechanisms of action. The fundamental concept upon which these models are based is that drugs bind with intracellular macromolecular receptors by means of ionic bonds, hydrogen bonds, and other electrostatic forces. Such a reversible combination is thought to form a drug-receptor complex of sufficient stability to alter the physiological response of the target system, consequently producing the observed pharmacological effect.

PHARMACOKINETICS

Anyone utilizing routine therapeutic drug monitoring as a guide to adjusting a patient's therapeutic regimen must constantly keep in mind that the plasma concentration achieved and maintained following the administration of a fixed drug dosage is a direct consequence of the interactions of a wide variety of interrelated processes (see Fig. 3-1), including drug absorption, distribution, metabolism, and excretion, and the physiological status of the patient. The study of these interrelationships forms the basis of pharmacokinetics.

Pharmacokinetics is the study of the time-course of drug and metabolite concentrations in different fluids, tissues, and excreta of the body, and of the mathematical relationships that can be utilized to develop models for interpretation and prediction of the drug concentration patterns observed in a given patient (Table 3-2). In the practical sense, pharmacokinetics as a discipline represents an attempt to utilize mathematical models to predict the distribution and excretion patterns of drugs, usually at steady-state concentrations, in response to a given dosage regimen. Applied clinical pharmacokinetics can be used in the clinical management of patients receiving a given drug. However, it is essential that the clinician recognize the theoretical limitations of pharmacokinetic models. For example, many models do not take into account multiple drug therapy or the clinical status of the patient. Interactions between drugs can alter the kinetics of each drug administered and thus affect plasma drug concentrations as well. Therefore, unless specific clinical data from a given patient are available, these models should be used only as a general guideline.

Table 3-2. General Factors Influencing Interpretation of Assay Data or Therapeutic Drug Monitoring

---

Patient compliance, including dosage error and wrong medication
Absorption via route of administration
Drug distribution
Biotransformation
Excretion
Genetic variability
Pathophysiological factors (acute or chronic disease)
Drug interactions
Drug tolerance
Inappropriate drug effects

The development of pharmacokinetics as a discipline was a direct consequence of the availability of techniques for monitoring drug levels in biological fluids and the attempts of investigators to correlate a given dosage of drug (mg/kg) with the observed plasma concentration and clinical response in large patient populations. The fundamental assumption of these studies was that the patient was at a steady state (i.e., the intake of a drug had been constant over a period of time, and drug elimination, as reflected in the rates of drug metabolism and excretion, was also constant). Based upon data derived from these studies, a number of computer programs have been developed that, given plasma concentration data with respect to time, will calculate the drug dosage necessary to achieve any specified plasma drug concentration in a specific patient. Unfortunately, these programs and the information derived from them are not yet widely available to practicing clinicians or clinical chemistry laboratories.

The clinical application of these programs and information does not require a detailed knowledge of pharmacokinetics. However, an awareness of the terminology and of fundamental principles is essential.

First-Order Kinetics

Any process associated with drug utilization exhibits first-order kinetics when there is a linear relationship between plasma drug concentration and total daily dose (mg/kg). Figure 3-3 (curve A) graphically depicts that an increase in the drug dose would be expected to result in a proportionate increase in plasma drug concentrations.

Zero-Order Kinetics

When the rate of a process is independent of concentration, it is said to follow zero-order kinetics. Zero-order kinetics become clearly apparent when a point is reached at which all of a drug's protein-binding sites are occupied, and/or drug excretion is occurring at a maximal rate. When a given drug utilization system is operating at its maximal rate, it is by definition *saturated*. Whereas plotting of drug plasma concentration versus total daily dose (mg/kg) initially yields an apparently straight line indicative of first-order kinetics, a sharp upward bend in the curve is seen as the saturation point is reached. The marked changes in drug clearance rates that occur beyond the saturation point, as represented by the disproportionate increase in plasma drug concentration following a given dosage increment, are the hallmark of zero-order kinetics (Fig. 3-3, curve B).

Fortunately, in clinical practice, only a few drugs exhibit zero-order kinetics. For most drugs, the plasma concentrations achieved at therapeutic dosage are low relative to the concentration necessary to saturate the par-

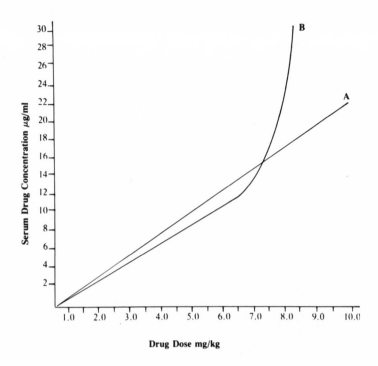

FIG. 3-3. (A) Dose-response curve for a drug observing first-order kinetics (linear). **(B)** Dose-response curve for a drug observing zero-order kinetics (nonlinear or saturation).

ticular system involved. Therefore, first-order kinetics are observed throughout the therapeutic range. There are notable exceptions to this rule, however, because both phenytoin and tricyclic antidepressants exhibit saturation kinetics near the upper limits of their respective therapeutic ranges. For any drug that exhibits zero-order kinetics, a very small dosage increment may result in a clinically significant elevation of plasma concentrations. It is to be noted that even though the initial dose-response curve may appear linear in drugs with zero-order kinetics, the drug clearance rate is altered throughout the dosage range and at all plasma concentrations and does not parallel the kinetics observed in a first-order relationship. It is for this reason that the half-life of phenytoin is different at any given plasma concentration. Although we commonly state that the half-life of phenytoin is 24 hours in reality, phenytoin half-life is concentration dependent (i.e., the higher the phenytoin concentration, the longer the half-life [Table 3-3]).

Drug Half-Life

Drug half-life is also referred to as the elimination half-time ($t_{1/2}$). It is the time required for elimination of half the concentration of a drug pres-

Table 3-3. Zero-Order Kinetic Predictions of Phenytoin Plasma Concentrations in a Hypothetical Patient[a]

Hours after last dose	Expected PHT level (μg/ml)	Half-life (hours)
6	36	75
12	32	67
18	28	60
24	24	53
30	21	46
36	17	40
42	14	33
48	10	27
54	7	22
60	5	17
66	3	14
72	1	11

[a]The computer-predicted phenytoin (PHT) blood levels listed are calculated for a male aged 40, weighing 70 kg and 175.3 cm tall at the time phenytoin dosage was discontinued. Blood level prediction following the initial phenytoin blood level is 40.0 μg/ml and absorption is assumed to be complete.

ent in the system, provided no additional drug is administered following a given point in time. For example, if the concentration of carbamazepine ($t_{1/2}$ = 18 hours) was 12 μg/ml, the time required to clear the drug to a concentration of 6 μg/ml would be 18 hours, provided no additional doses of the drug had been given. It must be emphasized that drug half-life is, in reality, a reflection of the individual rates of the several different processes that regulate drug clearance. The clearance rate (i.e., the rates of drug metabolism and excretion) is the primary determinant of the drug half-life in any given patient.

Fate of a Single Drug Dose

Following the administration of a single drug dose, a peak plasma concentration is reached when the absorption phase is almost complete (Fig. 3-4). The plasma concentration then begins to decline, even as the drug remaining in the intestine continues to be absorbed. The rate of this decline in the plasma concentration is dependent upon the rates of absorption, metabolism, and excretion of the drug. Once the absorption phase is complete, the rate of decline in the plasma concentration is a reflection of the clearance (elimination) rate, which is the sum of the rates of excre-

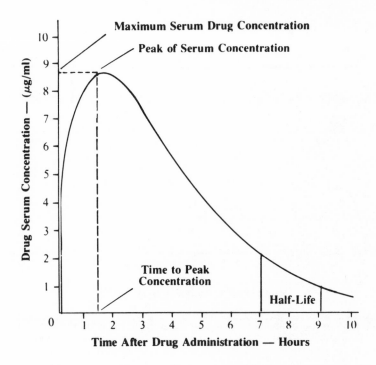

FIG. 3-4. Dose-response curve after the oral administration of a single dose of a hypothetical drug.

tion and metabolism of the drug. Following completion of the absorption phase, the half-life can be determined by measuring the decline in the plasma concentration over fixed time intervals.

Steady State

When long-term oral therapy is initiated, the drug will continue to accumulate within the body until such time as the rate of clearance, which comprises all tissue distribution, metabolic, and excretion processes involved in drug disposition, equals the rate of administration. When the equilibrium between drug clearance and intake is achieved, the system is said to be a *steady state* (i.e., the amount of drug ingested over a 24-hour period is equal to the amount of drug eliminated in the same 24-hour period). Over a period of time, body and plasma drug concentrations will increase exponentially until they reach a steady state or plateau (Fig. 3-5). It requires seven half-lives of drug administration before a true steady-state concentration is achieved and stabilized. Steady processes are, however, 97% complete within five half-lives and as a practical rule of thumb, five times the half-life of any drug is the time required to achieve a steady

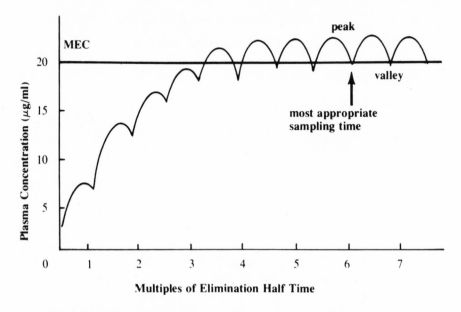

FIG. 3-5. Dose-response curve following repeated oral drug administration. MEC, minimum effective concentration.

state. For example, carbamazepine, which has a half-life of 18 hours, requires a period of 18×5 or 90 hours (4 days) to achieve a steady state. In contrast, drugs with short half-lives such as primidone or valproate, which usually have half-lives of 6–8 hours, require only 33–44 hours to reach a steady state whereas phenobarbital, which has a half-life of 4 days requires 28 days to reach a full steady state. Table 3-4 lists the percentage of the final steady-state drug concentration that is achieved at each half-life interval.

Table 3-4. Percentage of Steady-State Plasma Levels Achieved at Each Half-Life Interval

Number of half-lives	Steady-state levels (%)
1	50
2	75
3	88
4	94
5	97
6	98
7	99

It is important to note that the same principles that govern the gradual accumulation of a drug to a steady state also apply when drug therapy is discontinued. For instance, if plasma phenobarbital is at a steady-state concentration and drug administration is stopped, there will be a period of 28 days, or seven half-lives, before the drug is completely eliminated from the body. This is why drugs with prolonged half-lives can still be detected in plasma for weeks or months after administration of the last dose. Bromides, with a half-life of 12 days, require 66 days for complete elimination (or to reach steady state). Desethylamiodarone, an active metabolite of the antiarrhythmic drug amiodarone has a half-life of 60 days thus requiring a year to reach steady state. An even more important concept is that *principles which govern achievement of steady state apply anytime a drug dose is changed* regardless of whether the dose is increased or decreased.

Plasma concentrations for drugs with first-order kinetics are linearly related to dose. For any change of dosage, after a steady state has been achieved, the principles regulating the time required to achieve a new steady-state stage still apply. To illustrate this important principle, if the maintenance dose of a drug was doubled, the new steady-state concentration would not double until the completion of seven half-lives. If a plasma drug concentration is determined before achievement of a new steady state, for example, after two half-lives, it will not reflect the true steady-state concentration of the drug. It is important to understand that, for drugs exhibiting zero-order kinetics, half-lives increase after the saturation point is reached. That is to say, after saturation, it will still take seven half-lives to reach steady state, but each half-life will be longer. This is why a phenytoin level of 35–40 μg/ml will not drop to 17–20 μg/ml 24 hours after the drug is discontinued: at these higher levels saturation of metabolic processes occurs, resulting in a half-life longer than 24 hours (see Table 3-2).

It is also essential to understand that the *full therapeutic effect of a given drug dose is not achieved until steady-state concentrations are reached.* Therefore, before a given dosage regimen is considered a failure, the clinician should be sure that steady-state concentrations have been achieved and maintained for an appropriate interval.

FACTORS THAT ALTER INDIVIDUAL DRUG DISPOSITION PATTERNS

Drug Absorption

Some patients receiving appropriate drug doses will have consistently low plasma drug concentrations. Generally, these patients are classified as either noncompliant or as fast drug metabolizers (see below). However, before classifying someone as a fast metabolizer, the patient's ability to absorb the administered drug should be evaluated. The distribution of drugs into tissues following parenteral administration is generally rapid and circumvents the problems associated with drug absorption following oral administration; however, most drugs are administered orally. Following oral administration, the type of drug preparation, drug solubility, concomitant administration of other drugs, whether or not the drug is taken with meals, the presence of diarrhea or constipation, and the clinical status of the patient can alter the amount of drug that will be absorbed from the gastrointestinal tract following a single dose (Fig. 3-6).

Malabsorption of an orally administered drug can often be confirmed by measuring serial plasma drug concentrations at given time intervals after parenteral administration of the prescribed dose. If altered absorption is present, the maximum plasma concentrations and observed drug half-life following the intravenous dose will be significantly higher than those achieved following the same dose administered orally. Conversely, if the patient's problem is fast drug metabolism, there will be no significant differences in the plasma concentrations achieved or the observed half-life regardless of the route of administration.

Drug Plasma Protein Binding and Free Drug Concentrations

The clinical utility of monitoring free drug concentrations is clearly established. The following outline is designed to draw your attention to some of the factors that can alter the interpretation of free drug concentration reports. Numerous reviews describing the general principles of drug-protein binding, the various psychological and pharmacological factors which can alter free drug concentrations, and the clinical implications of free drug concentrations are available.

One of the underlying tenets of clinical pharmacology is *only the free drug is pharmacologically active.* Only free drugs can cross biological membranes to interact with a given receptor to alter its function (by interaction with the receptor, we really mean the interaction of the drug with any biochemical or physiological system to increase, decrease, or maintain the function of that system at a given level). The following general principles should always be borne in mind with respect to free and total drug concentrations.

1. An equilibrium exists between total drug concentration and free drug concentration in plasma and tissues.

2. For most drugs, a specific fraction of the total drug present in plasma is bound to plasma proteins.

3. The amount of any given drug bound to proteins depends upon that drug's physiochemical properties with respect to those of the protein

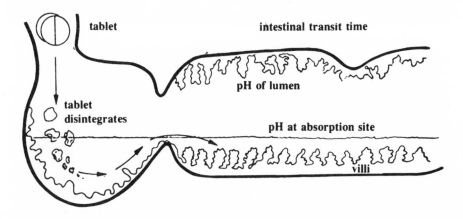

FIG. 3-6. Factors affecting drug absorption.

to which it binds. Binding of drugs to protein occurs by electrostatic interactions, between the ionic changes of the drug and protein and hydrogen bonding. Drugs are not covalently bound to proteins under normal physiological conditions.

4. Figure 3-1 illustrates the interrelationships between total and free drug concentration in plasma, extracellular fluid, and tissue. It is clearly evident that any change in the total drug concentration will be reflected by a change in the absolute free drug concentration as the equilibrium adjusts. Changes in free drug concentration in plasma water will result in a new equilibration of the drug concentrations in extracellular fluid and tissues. Thus, ultimately the tissue drug concentrations will either increase or decrease following a change in the total drug concentration.

5. Because of this equilibrium, a general rule of thumb is that the total concentration of a drug in plasma reflects the free drug concentration.

6. A decrease in the concentration of a plasma protein to which a drug is bound will result in an increase in the free drug fraction even though the total drug concentration remains unchanged.

7. An increase in the plasma protein concentration to which a drug is bound will result in a decrease in the free drug concentration even though the total drug concentration remains unchanged.

8. Changes in drug protein binding occur under certain normal physiological states: (a) Fetal albumin present in newborn infants has less binding affinity for acidic drugs than does albumin in infants or children. Thus, free drug concentrations in neonates are slightly (3–5%) higher than those observed in children or adults with the same total drug concentration. (b) Pregnancy results in decreased drug binding to albumin. (c) Individuals over 65 years of age tend to have decreased plasma albu-

min concentrations. Consequently, increased free drug concentrations are present at total drug concentrations that would normally be considered optimal. Thus, it is possible for the elderly to present with clinical signs of drug intoxication secondary to elevated free drug concentration in the presence of therapeutic concentrations. (e) Any physiological factor which results in an increased protein concentration (hyperalbuminemia) will result in a decreased free drug concentration. (f) Any physiological factor which results in a decreased protein concentration (hypoalbuminemia) will result in an increased free drug concentration.

9. Disease states which alter physiological function can alter the amount of a drug bound to plasma proteins. *Renal failure:* The elevation of serum creatinine and blood urea nitrogen (BUN) associated with renal failure results in a blockade of the secondary drug-binding sites. The drug-binding capacity of the primary albumin drug-binding sites does not appear altered in renal failure. It is believed that alteration of secondary binding sites is a consequence of the carbamylation of sulfhydryl groups by the cyanate released during the spontaneous decomposition of urea to cyanate and ammonia. Under these circumstances, one would expect to see increased free drug fractions. A good rule of thumb is that patients in renal failure receiving drugs which are bound to albumin show a free fraction that is usually no more than twice as great as that which would be seen in the same individual under normal physiological conditions. For example, the normal free fraction of phenytoin is 0.10. In patients with renal failure, the phenytoin free fraction is usually 0.20–0.25.

10. Basic drugs including tricyclic antidepressants are bound primarily to α_1-acid-glycoprotein (α_1AGp) (orosomucoid). α_1AGp is an acute phase-reactant protein whose plasma concentrations are significantly increased in response to altered physiological states. Elevated α_1AGp concentrations associated with myocardial infarction, infection, cancer, and immunological disease are well documented. As the concentration of α_1AGp increases, the number of sites able to bind basic drugs also increases. Under these circumstances, the free basic drug concentration will decrease during an acute phase reaction. Basic free drug concentrations are often suboptimal even though the total drug concentration is optimal or even at toxic levels.

It is important to bear in mind that other disease processes, particularly myocardial infarction can dramatically alter free drug concentrations. Myocardial infarctions represent a separate issue. The binding of acidic drugs is not significantly altered by myocardial infarctions. However, the binding of basic drugs including tricyclic antidepressants can be significantly altered by a myocardial infarction. It is always to be remembered that following a myocardial infarction, there is an increase in the concentrations of α_1AGp. The elevation of α_1AGp following a myocardial infarction occurs over a period of several days; however, the initial significant increases in α_1AGp concentrations occur within the first 24 hours following an infarction. After the initial infarction, the patient will experience further rises in α_1AGp over a period of 2–7 days. Following this final α_1AGp rise, there is again a decrease in α_1AGp levels over a period of 12–14 days to their preinfarction values. Thus, following a myocardial infarction there is a period of approximately 24–30 days when the α_1AGp concentrations are elevated and binding of basic drugs is abnormal.

The interpretation and clinical application of total drug concentrations to patient management during an actual phase reaction can be complex. When interpreting free or total basic drug concentrations, the following principles must always be followed: (1) Assess the clinical status of the patient in relation to the desired therapeutic goals. (2) Always remember that an acute phase elevation of α_1AGp is characterized by a rise to maximum concentrations which may be two to three times base-line concentrations. (3) The initial α_1AGp elevation begins within 12 hours of the reaction and may not peak for several days. (4) As the patient's physiological state returns to normal, the α_1AGp concentrations will also return to normal over a period of days. (5) As the α_1AGp returns to normal, the number of basic drug-binding sites decreases and the free drug concentration increases. If basic drug dosages were increased during the acute phase reaction, the patient may develop clinical signs of drug intoxication at a total plasma concentration that had previously not produced side effects. Basic drugs are bound primarily to α_1AGp. Thus, the increase in levels observed of α_1AGp following a myocardial infarction result in increased binding and decreased free levels. Consequently, it is quite possible that a patient maintained at a therapeutic concentration of a basic drug such as lidocaine, procainamide, or quinidine for the management of arrhythmias associated with a myocardial infarction, may in reality exhibit subtherapeutic-free lidocaine concentrations. The same rules apply to the tricyclic antidepressants or other basic drugs which are also bound to α_1AGp used in the management of various disease processes.

11. A good rule of thumb is that the greater the affinity of the drug for a binding protein, the more apt it is to displace a drug which has less affinity for the same protein from its protein-binding sites. When a patient is receiving multiple drug therapy, it is highly probable that there will be a marked difference between the protein-binding affinity of two simultaneously administered drugs. If the drugs compete for the same binding sites, either on albumin or on α_1AGp, the more weakly bound drug will be displaced from its binding site. The displaced drug may be more rapidly cleared or metabolized; in these situations the free concentration of the displaced drug will be lower. If the initial displaced free concentrations are high enough, the actual free concentrations may rise secondary to saturation (zero-order) kinetics of the clearance pathways. A good example of the variable effects of displacement of one drug by an-

other are the free-drug concentration changes associated with the coadministration of phenytoin and valproic acid. Phenytoin is 90% protein bound and valproic acid is 95% protein bound. Valproic acid has a greater affinity for the albumin-binding sites than does phenytoin. Therefore, in a patient receiving phenytoin who is placed on valproic acid, the valproic acid will displace the phenytoin from its protein-binding sites. If the free phenytoin concentration is less than 1.7 μg/ml, the end result will be an enhanced clearance of phenytoin which will result in a decrease in both the total and the free phenytoin concentrations. Under these circumstances, it is possible for the patient's total phenytoin level to decrease by half within 24 hours after placing him on valproic acid. Conversely, if the patient's free phenytoin concentration is 1.7 or above and the patient is placed on valproic acid, the saturation kinetics of phenytoin will be exceeded, the displaced free phenytoin will accumulate to toxic levels (2.5–3.0 μg/ml), and the total levels will also increase to 25–30 μg/ml. This is because the clearance of phenytoin is saturated. This phenomena can occur even in the presence of what would normally be considered to be optimal phenytoin levels (i.e., total phenytoin concentrations between 18 and 20 mg/ml). Under these circumstances, one would expect to see clinical signs of phenytoin intoxication in the presence of an elevated free phenytoin concentration. The criteria we have described above for phenytoin apply equally as well to the coadministration of other antiepileptic drugs and valproic acid.

Drug Metabolism

Any foreign compound that enters the body is considered a toxin which must be eliminated. Drug elimination mechanisms become more complex as one proceeds up the phylogenetic scale from fish to man. There is a progressive increase in the ability of the body to chemically alter foreign compounds into compounds that are more water-soluble and less fat-soluble. The more water-soluble a compound, the more readily it is excreted. It is generally believed that the unique efficiency of the liver to metabolize drugs evolved as a mechanism for detoxifying poisonous substances ingested with food.

The drug-metabolizing enzymes of the liver interact with a wide variety of chemical structures. Metabolites of many drugs are conjugated within the liver to either glucuronic acid, amino acids, or sulfates, thus increasing water solubility even more and, consequently, the rate of renal excretion. For example, p-hydroxyphenytoin, the major metabolite of phenytoin, is conjugated with glucuronic acid. This conjugation increases its water solubility almost 100 times.

Most drug metabolism takes place within the microsomal fraction of the hepatocyte. The microsomal enzyme systems are also responsible for the metabolism of endogenous steroids. These systems are not designed to recognize specific drugs; rather, they act upon classes of compounds with similar structures. The same enzymes that are responsible for the hydroxylation of phenytoin may also hydroxylate other drugs containing an appropriate phenyl ring. Therefore, when phenytoin is administered simultaneously with one of these drugs, there may be clinically significant alterations of drug concentrations as a direct consequence of competition for metabolic sites. Clinically, one would expect to see higher serum concentrations of the drug with the least affinity for the enzyme. Phenytoin has a very low affinity for microsomal enzymes. Thus, administration of a drug with a greater affinity for the enzyme than phenytoin will decrease phenytoin's rate of metabolism, and plasma phenytoin concentrations will increase. One should realize, however, that not all compounds are metabolized at the same site. One can be a fast metabolizer of one group of compounds and normally metabolize others. Similarly, one compound may displace phenytoin from its metabolic site whereas another will have no effect.

One characteristic of the hepatic microsomal system is that it can be induced to metabolize drugs at a faster rate. As increasing amounts of a drug are administered, the body, in its attempt to eliminate the drug, synthesizes new proteins in the form of enzymes capable of metabolizing that agent. Increased activity of drug-metabolizing enzymatic systems is not necessarily induced with every dosage increment or with the addition of another drug to the patient's regimen. There is a maximum rate at which protein synthesis can occur. Thus, if a patient has been regularly receiving a drug with known enzyme-induction properties, it does not follow that a second drug of similar structure added to the patient's therapeutic regimen will cause a marked increase in the rate of metabolism of the first and second drug.

Genetic factors play a major role in determining the ability of a patient to metabolize drugs. Individuals of different ethnic origins as well as individuals in certain families metabolize drugs (e.g., phenytoin or isoniazid) at a faster or slower rate than the general population. A fast drug metabolizer will require a greater daily dose (mg/kg) than a normal individual to achieve the same serum concentration. Conversely, a slow drug metabolizer given standard drug dosages will invariably develop drug toxicity.

Absolute identification of fast and slow drug metabolizers depends upon the quantitative identification of urinary drug-metabolite excretion profiles as well as on the serial determination of plasma drug concentrations. Generally, plasma drug concentrations of slow metabolizers will be significantly higher than would be observed in the general population receiving the same mg/kg/day dosage. Consistently high plasma concentrations on normal or low drug doses is suggestive of slow drug metabolism, although a drug interaction or disease process that blocks drug metabolism will also result in elevated plasma concentrations. On the other hand, fast drug metabolizers usually exhibit consistently low plasma concentrations on standard dosage regimens. Because plasma drug levels in noncompliant patients mimic those observed in fast metabolizers, there is a tendency to identify noncompliant patients as fast metabolizers. Use of plasma drug concentrations alone to identify fast and slow metabolizers can be misleading. Metabolite urinary excretion patterns help to clarify whether a given patient's plasma drug levels are caused by metabolic alterations, noncompliance, or another problem.

Generally, drugs are metabolized from pharmacologically active agents to inactive products, incapable of eliciting a given therapeutic response. For example, the addition of sodium valproate to the regimen of a patient who is receiving phenytoin may result in a marked decrease in total phenytoin concentrations. This decrease is a direct consequence of the displacement of phenytoin from its plasma protein-binding sites. The displaced phenytoin is rapidly converted to its inactive metabolite, p-hydroxyphenytoin. The observed fall in total phenytoin levels is indicative of an altered rate of phenytoin disposition.

There are exceptions to this rule: Some drug metabolites have a greater biological activity than the parent compound. For example, diazepam is rapidly metabolized to desmethyldiazepam (nordiazepam), which is the most active antianxiety agent of all the diazepam metabolites. As a general rule, when a compound has a less polar-active metabolite, the half-life of the active metabolite is significantly longer than that of the parent compound. Such is the case with procainamide and N-acetylprocainamide (NAPA). The half-life of procainamide is 3–4 hours, whereas NAPA has a half-life of 6–9 hours in patients with normal creatinine clearance. This means that there will be an accumulation of NAPA, the active metabolite, within the system and at its site of action. It is to be emphasized that most immunoassay techniques used for routine therapeutic drug monitoring today measure the parent compound and do not measure drug metabolites.

The clinical status of a patient can also dramatically alter drug utilization patterns. Hepatitis can impair drug metabolism. If the liver has lost its reserve capacity, patients with hepatitis can become severely intoxicated when given drugs dependent upon hepatic degradation. Congestive heart failure can significantly alter the distribution of drugs to tissues, thus precipitating altered drug utilization and response patterns.

Renal Excretion

Urinary excretion is the major pathway for the elimination of drugs and their metabolites. For any drug that is not extensively metabolized (e.g., antibiotics), changes in renal function will alter that drug's plasma concentrations. If renal function is impaired, drug plasma concentrations can become elevated.

Uremic patients and those with congestive heart failure have decreased renal drug clearance. Interestingly, drug metabolites are so water-soluble that a significant decrease in urinary output will not by itself result in increased plasma concentrations of most conjugated drug metabolites.

Patient Noncompliance

It has been suggested that 60–70% of all patients do not take their medications in the manner prescribed by their physicians. The most common cause of suboptimal drug concentrations, and consequent failure to achieve the desired therapeutic response, is patient noncompliance. Whenever a patient presents with consistently low plasma drug concentrations, noncompliance should be considered the probable cause. Noncompliance can usually be demonstrated by careful supervision of the patient's daily drug intake over a specified time interval (usually five half-lives of the drug) with routine monitoring of serum drug concentrations at appropriate intervals. If there is a progressive increase in serum drug concentration over the time interval selected, the patient has been noncompliant.

The administration of the recommended or average total daily dose of a given drug without taking into account the numerous factors that alter drug disposition in each patient can also lead to consistently low serum drug concentrations. Thus, if the serum concentrations remain low under supervised intake, other causes such as drug malabsorption or rapid drug metabolism should be suspected. Failure to individualize drug therapy (physician noncompliance) is frequently the cause for suboptimal drug concentrations.

PHARMACOGENETIC ALTERATIONS OF DRUG DISPOSITION IN HEALTHY INDIVIDUALS ARE COMMON

As noted above, drug clearance is significantly regulated by genetic factors. In a large population of patients, one could predict that if the entire population were given the same mg/kg dosage of a drug, there would be marked differences in the ability of individuals within the population to utilize the drug. These genetic differences will be reflected by a marked variability of the steady-state plasma concentrations observed in this population.

For example, in a population of patients receiving phenytoin at a standard therapeutic dose of 5 mg/kg/day, one would theoretically expect all patients to have a therapeutic drug level of 15 μg/ml. In reality, plasma concentrations will range from 0 μg/ml, which suggests drug malabsorption, patient noncompliance, or fast drug metabolism, to levels of 40–50 μg/ml, which may indicate drug interactions, patients who have hepatic or renal disease, or patients who are genetically slow drug metabolizers.

As an example, consider the incidence of fast and slow metabolism in patients receiving isoniazid, a drug commonly used in the treatment of tuberculosis whose primary metabolic pathway is acetylation. Approximately 40% of all Caucasians are rapid acetylators of isoniazid. In contrast, over 90% of Japanese and Eskimos are rapid acetylators. This genetic variability requires individualization of therapeutic regimens to assure the maintenance of optimal isoniazid concentrations in the different ethnic populations and individuals within a given ethnic population. The same rules hold in these populations for other drugs (e.g., procainamide) which are acetylated.

PATIENT INFORMATION NECESSARY FOR INTERPRETATION OF DRUG CONCENTRATIONS

Wide individual variability exists in patient utilization of drugs as a direct consequence of genetic factors, multiple drug therapy, age, and weight (Table 3-5). Successful TDM is based on individualization of drug therapy based upon assessing the significance of the plasma concentration, the clinical status of the patient, and the therapeutic goals. In order to derive as much information as possible about the pharmacological status of the patient, each clinician utilizing TDM as a guide for regulating a patient's therapeutic regimen should have the following information available at the time any drug is monitored.

Patient age. It is clearly established there are marked age-dependent differences in drug utilization, in particular the transition ages between neonate and infant, child and adolescent, and adult and geriatric.

Patient weight. The weight of the patient is essential for mathematical calculations of the relationships among the drug dose, plasma concentration, and drug clearance. Any factor that alters drug half-life (clearance) will alter the drug's steady-state concentration. During multiple drug therapy, two drugs may compete for the same metabolic site. This com-

Table 3-5. Information Needed for Interpretation of Drug Levels

Patient age, weight, and sex
List of all of the drugs that the patient is receiving
Total daily dose of all drugs
Dosage regimen and dosage form of each drug
Time the last dose of drug, the level of which is being requested, was administered
Clinical status of the patient
Time the specimen was drawn

petition will decrease the rate of metabolism of the drug that is excluded from the site and prolong its half-life. Because the half-life is prolonged (clearance is decreased), a new, higher steady-state drug concentration will be achieved and maintained, as long as the multiple drug therapy is continued.

All drugs that the patient is receiving. Knowledge of the drugs that the patient is receiving, in addition to the agent being monitored, is essential for identification of potential drug interactions that might alter plasma concentrations as well as for the identification of compounds that may interfere with a given analytical technique. In addition, multiple drug therapy can also alter absorption, protein binding, and renal clearance of a given agent. Change in any of these factors can result in altered steady-state concentrations.

Total daily dosage of drugs. A knowledge of the total daily dosage for each drug administered is necessary to mathematically determine the patient's total daily drug use in mg/kg. Without this information it is impossible to correlate the patient's actual plasma concentration with his expected plasma concentration based upon the prescribed drug dose. Knowledge of the mg/kg dose allows the prediction of the patient's expected plasma drug concentration using the appropriate mathematical formulas available in any pharmacology text. Predicted can then be correlated with the observed (measured) drug concentration to provide an indication of the patient's pharmacological status.

Clinical status of the patient. It is well established that acute or chronic disease can dramatically alter drug utilization patterns. Awareness of the patient's current clinical status is particularly important for regulation of drug therapy in patients with hepatitis or renal failure. Drug clearance is dramatically altered during renal and liver disease because the elimination rates of the drugs are changed. Consequently, new steady-state levels will be achieved that may differ significantly from those observed in healthy individuals. Without the knowledge of the clinical status of the patient, it is impossible for those interpreting drug concentrations to distinguish an altered drug utilization pattern that is associated with a given disease state from other factors (noncompliance, drug interactions, etc.) that can present with a similar pattern.

Critical time intervals. The time at which the last dose of drug was administered and the time at which the blood specimen was drawn are essential pieces of information. Without this information, it is difficult to assess whether the actual plasma concentration represents a peak or trough level. A knowledge of the actual sampling time and dosage interval is extremely important for accurate interpretation of plasma concentrations of drugs with short half-lives, such as primidone and valproic acid.

As a rule, specimens for TDM should be drawn at a trough (i.e., the time when the plasma concentration should be at its lowest level for that dosing interval). Measurement of peak concentrations following oral administration is difficult because of the marked individual variability in drug absorption patterns. Peak levels are indicated, however, in certain situations following intravenous drug administration and have been reported to be of value in the monitoring of antibiotics, theophylline, and certain antiarrhythmic drugs.

Selection of the time when a specimen is drawn in relation to drug administration should be based upon the pharmacokinetic properties of the drug and the dosage form. The patient should be at or near steady state when the sample is drawn. After any dosage adjustment, time should be allowed for equilibrium (i.e., a new steady state to be reestablished with the new dosage regimen) before another specimen is drawn. Specimens drawn immediately before administration of the next oral dose provide trough serum levels for drugs administered on a chronic basis; the trough level should ideally be above the minimum effective concentration level. Specimens for peak levels are generally drawn 15–30 minutes after intravenous administration, 1–2 hours after intramuscular administration, and 1–5 hours after oral administration (depending on the rate of drug absorption and distribution). When the specimen is going to be drawn during an infusion, the sample should be taken from the opposite limb.

Anyone involved in the interpretation of information derived from therapeutic drug monitoring must always bear in mind that their *interpretation of plasma drug concentrations must always be carried out in conjunction with an assessment of the clinical status of the patient!* Rather than therapeutic ranges, the clinician should be concerned with optimal concentrations. The optimal concentration of a drug is defined as that concentration of drug present in plasma or some other biological fluid or tissue that provides the desired therapeutic response in most patients. It is to be emphasized that the severity of the disease process determines the amount of drug necessary to achieve a given therapeutic effect. Thus, it is quite possible that a given patient may achieve the desired therapeutic effect at a plasma concentration well below the population optimal range. Others may require levels above those usually considered optimal to achieve the desired clinical effect and may tolerate these levels without evidence for toxicity. Still others will not achieve the desired therapeutic effect even when plasma concentrations are elevated into the toxic range. If the desired therapeutic effect is achieved at usually suboptimal plasma concentrations, there is no reason to increase the dose of medication in that patient. Conversely, in a patient who does not achieve the desired effect at a suboptimal plasma level, the dose of that drug should be increased. Every attempt should be made to avoid the prescription of additional drugs simply to increase the plasma concentration into what is commonly referred to as the therapeutic range. Obviously, the interpretation of plasma drug concentrations must take into account the various factors that can alter the steady-state plasma concentration achieved on a given dosage regimen.

DETERMINING DOSAGE INTERVALS

Generally, in order to maintain a smooth, constant steady-state drug concentration, without excessive fluctuations, dosage intervals should be less than half of each particular drug's half-life. To illustrate this in practical terms, phenytoin would be given every 12 hours because its half-life is 24 hours, whereas valproate would be given every 3 hours, because its half-life is 6–8 hours.

Short dosage intervals (3–4 hours) are often impractical in outpatients, but drugs with short lives should be administered at least once each half-life. The fundamental concept is to maintain the trough drug concentration within the desired range (i.e., above the minimum effect concentration), while avoiding peak concentrations that reach toxic levels (i.e., exceed the minimum toxic concentration). As long as the dosage schedule and the interval between peak and trough concentrations of drugs are maintained during the dosage interval, an appropriate steady-state concentration will be maintained. If the dosage interval is too long relative to the half-life of the drug, the plasma concentration just prior to the next dose may be insufficient to provide the desired therapeutic effect. For example, a patient whose phenytoin level falls from 14 to 9 μg/ml may have a seizure at the lower level but not at the higher one. For any drug, it is possible to maintain a plasma concentration within the optimal therapeutic range at all times by adhering to an appropriate dosage schedule.

If a patient's drug absorption is very rapid, or if dosage intervals are excessively short, he may experience periods of drug intoxication that may present clinically with symptoms appropriate for that drug. These symptoms usually appear transiently and at fixed intervals following drug administration. The toxicity is attributed to a peak plasma concentration above the minimal toxic concentration shortly after drug administration. Such side effects can often be eliminated by increasing the dosage interval or decreasing the dose given in order to assure that peak concentrations are not excessive.

MONITORING STEADY-STATE DRUG CONCENTRATIONS

When long-term oral therapy is initiated, the drug will continue to accumulate within the body until such time as the rate of drug clearance (elimination) is in equilibrium with the total daily drug intake. At this time, steady state is achieved. We again emphasize that the time required to reach a stabilized steady state is seven half-lives following institution of drug therapy or alteration of total daily dose, although steady-state processes are 97% complete within five half-lives. It is possible, if one knows the time of initiation of drug therapy, to extrapolate predicted steady-state plasma concentrations by correcting for the number of half-lives ex-

Table 3-6. Antiepileptic Drug Pharmacokinetic Data

AED	Half-life (hours)	Time to steady-state (days)	V_D(L/kg)	% Bioavail-ability (oral)	% Protein binding	Optimal plasma concentration (μg/ml)
Phenytoin	10–34[a]	7–28	0.6–8.0	90–95	90	10–20[a]
Phenobarbital	46–136	14–21	0.6	90–100	50	20–40
Primidone	3.3–19	1–4	0.43–1.1	90–100	80	8–12
Carbamazepine	12 if monotherapy; 5–14 if poly-therapy	21–28 for complete autoinduction	1–2	>75	40–90	8–12
Valproic acid	8–20	1–3	0.1–0.5	100	95[b]	80–100
Ethosuximide	50–70	6–12	0.67	90–100	0	80–100

[a]Exhibits saturation (zero-order) kinetics. Half-life varies with plasma concentration.
[b]Protein binding saturates at approximately 100 μg/ml.

Table 3-7. Antidepressant Drug Pharmacokinetic Data[a]

Antidepressants	Half-life (hours)	Time to steady-state (days)	V_D(L/kg)	% Bioavail-ability (oral)	% Protein binding	Optimal plasma concentration (ng/ml)
Tertiary amines						
Amitriptyline	10–22	5–7	12–16	37–59	95	60–220[b]
Doxepin	11–23	5–7	12–28	17–37	NE	30–150[b]
Imipramine	11–25	5–7	15–31	19–35	95	100–300[b]
Secondary amines						
Protriptyline	67–89	21–28	21–23	77–93	92	100–200
Nortriptyline	18–44	5–10	14–22	46–56	92	50–150
Desipramine	12–24	5–7	26–42	51	90	40–160
Other agents						
Amoxapine	8–30	4–7	NE	NE	90	180[b]
Fluoxetine	24–72	5–12	12–97	100	94	NE
Maprotiline	27–57	5–12	23	37	88	200–300
Trazodone	10–12	2–4	NE	NE	92	NE

[a]NE, not established.
[b]Parent compound plus active metabolite.

pired before sampling. This technique, however, provides only a rough estimate of the expected steady-state concentrations.

Remember, the pharmacological activity of the drug may be eliminated even though the drug's metabolite is still present in the body. A sudden change in measured steady-state drug concentrations usually serves as an indicator of altered drug disposition of the pharmacologically active (parent) compound.

For example, the addition of sodium valproate to the regimen of a patient who is receiving phenytoin may result in a marked decrease in total phenytoin concentrations. This decrease is a direct consequence of the displacement of phenytoin from its plasma protein-binding sites. The displaced phenytoin is rapidly converted to its inactive metabolite: *p*-hydroxyphenytoin. The observed fall in total phenytoin levels is indicative of an altered rate of phenytoin disposition.

The pharmacokinetic profiles of the antiepileptic drugs and the antidepressant drugs presented in Tables 3-6 and 3-7 represent general guidelines. It must be remembered that individual patients have their own profiles, which are determined by all the factors discussed above.

SUGGESTED READING

Avery GS, ed. *Drug Treatment: Principles and Practice of Clinical Pharmacology and Therapeutics*, 2nd ed. Sydney: ADIS, 1980.

Gerson B, Anhalt JP. *High-Pressure Liquid Chromatography and Therapeutic Drug Monitoring.* Chicago: American Association of Clinical Pathology, 1980.

Gilman AG, Goodman LS, Gilman A. *The Pharmacological Basis of Therapeutics,* 6th ed. New York: Macmillan, 1980.

Maggio ET, ed. *Enzyme Immunoassay.* Boca Raton: CRC Press, 1980.

Melmon KL, Morelli HI, eds. *Clinical Pharmacology: Basic Principles in Therapeutics,* 2nd ed. New York: Macmillan, 1978.

Morselli PL, ed. *Drug Disposition During Development.* New York: Spectrum Publ., 1977.

Morselli PL, Pippenger CE, Penry JK, eds. *Antiepileptic Drug Therapy in Pediatrics.* New York: Raven Press, 1983.

Moyer TP. Practical therapeutic drug monitoring. In: Homburger HA, Batsakis JG, eds. *Clinical Laboratory Annual,* Vol. 2. Norwalk: Appleton-Century-Crofts, 1982: 279–322.

Pippenger CE. Pediatric clinical pharmacology of antiepileptic drugs: a special consideration. In: Pippenger CE, Penry JK, Kutt H, eds. *Antiepileptic Drugs, Quantitative Analysis and Interpretation.* New York: Raven Press, 1977: 315–319.

Pippenger CE. *Principles of Therapeutic Drug Monitoring.* Palo Alto: Syva Monitor, Syva Company, 1981.

Pippenger CE, Penry JK, Kutt H, eds. Antiepileptic Drugs: Quantitative Analysis and Interpretation. New York: Raven Press, 1978.

Rowland M, Tozer TN. *Clinical Pharmacokinetics: Concepts and Application.* Philadelphia: Lea and Febiger, 1980.

Winter ME. *Basic Clinical Pharmacokinetics.* San Francisco: Applied Therapeutics, 1980.

Woodbury DM, Penry JK, Pippenger CE, eds. *Antiepileptic Drugs,* 2nd ed. New York: Raven Press, 1982.

4

Clinically Significant Antiepileptic Drug Interactions

C. E. Pippenger

The purpose of this chapter is to once again draw the attention of health care professionals to the many factors which can result in alteration of drug disposition and therefore drug concentrations during either acute or chronic drug therapy. This review is limited to commonly encountered drug interactions that are associated with antiepileptic drug therapy.

Three basic principles must always be remembered when considering drug interactions: (1) Drugs alter the activity of a physiological or biochemical system to return it as closely as possible to its normal level of activity. (2) The therapeutic regimens necessary to control many disease processes including the epilepsies and psychiatric disease often require multiple drug therapy. There is no such thing as a drug with only one pharmacological action, but rather drugs at any plasma or tissue concentration exert multiple effects upon different physiological systems. It is for this reason that patients receiving chronic drug therapy experience side effects even in the presence of the desired therapeutic effect and optimal drug concentrations. For example, it is now clearly recognized that the antiepileptic drugs, phenytoin, phenobarbital, and primidone at therapeutic plasma concentrations, impair cognitive function (see Chapter 7). (3) For most drugs there is a direct relationship between the plasma (tissue) concentrations and the observed therapeutic response. The higher the plasma concentration, the more probable it is that other physiological and/or biochemical systems will be affected in some manner by the drug, and clinical toxicity will develop. (4) One of the greatest misconceptions in therapeutic drug monitoring, however, is that such a linear relationship exists for all drugs; that is, that increasing the total dose brings about a concomitant and directly proportional increase in the plasma concentration. This is not the case. It must always be remembered that certain commonly prescribed drugs exhibit zero-order (saturation) kinetics. Certain drugs including phenytoin, nortriptyline, theophylline, and others demonstrate an apparently linear dose-concentration relationship only over a given range. Beyond this range, what would clinically be considered a negligible dosage increase produces a marked and completely disproportionate elevation of the plasma concentration that usually leads to adverse side effects.

The fundamental principles of applied clinical pharmacology and therapeutic drug monitoring have been extensively reviewed in Chapter 3. In summary, any drug may increase, decrease, or normalize the physiological function of tissues, organs, or body systems. The mechanism of action of a drug refers to the biochemical or physical process that initiates a biological response at a specific site. This response depends on a chemical interaction of a drug with a functionally viable component of some physiological system. However, because we still don't know the exact molecular mechanism of action for most drugs, theoretical models are utilized to explain them. The fundamental concept of these models is the existence of intracellular macromolecular receptors that, when stimulated, elicit a particular biological response. More specifically, we believe drugs combine reversibly with receptors by means of ionic bonds, hydrogen bonds, and van der Waal's forces. This combination forms a drug-receptor complex of sufficient stability to alter the physiological response of the target system and produce a given pharmacological effect as long as the drug concentrations at the receptor site are sufficiently high to activate the receptor.

Anything that changes the absorption, distribution, protein-binding metabolism, or excretion of a drug alters the plasma and tissue concentrations of a drug. If the plasma concentrations are increased under any of these circumstances, the desired therapeutic effects of a drug will not only be achieved but the probability of an increased incidence of adverse side effects is significantly enhanced. Conversely, if the plasma concentrations of a drug are decreased as a result of an alteration of any of these parameters, the probability that the desired therapeutic response will be achieved is significantly decreased and the probability of adverse drug interactions is significantly less.

Drug interactions can be classified into two types, idiosyncratic and drug–drug interactions. Drug–drug interactions are common and can occur in any patient, whereas idiosyncratic drug reactions are infrequent and occur only in those patients predisposed to develop them secondary to a specific drug exposure.

Our knowledge and understanding of which drug interactions are clinically significant constantly change. When introducing a new drug into the marketplace, one usually first encounters scattered case reports of drug interactions during the Phase II (efficacy) clinical trials as the drug is administered to a few hundred individuals. A greater incidence of reports is observed when the drug is in expanded Phase III (large population efficacy) clinical trials. The most common identification of drug interactions, however, occurs once a drug has reached the marketplace and is administered to a large patient population. Because no two people respond to a drug in exactly the same manner, it follows that the more people who receive a drug, the greater the probability of a drug interaction. Basically, clinical trials are designed to establish efficacy and safety. The ultimate goal of clinical trials is to prevent those drugs which would ultimately be inefficacious or highly toxic from reaching the marketplace.

IDIOSYNCRATIC DRUG INTERACTIONS

One of the major concerns about prescribing any new drug to a patient is the clinician's constant nagging fear that the drug will produce a severe idiosyncratic drug interaction. The clinical hallmark of idiosyncratic drug reactions is that they usually occur without any warning. There is no correlation between the patient's prior clinical status, drug dose, or plasma drug concentrations and the adverse reaction. It is generally accepted that idiosyncratic reactions are most likely to occur early during the course of a new drug therapy. Therefore, physicians are taught to be especially vigilant during the first few weeks or months following introduction of a new drug into the patient's regimen. However, an idiosyncratic reaction can occur at any time during the course of therapy. The hepatotoxicity or acute pancreatitis associated with valproic acid therapy has been reported to occur within 1 month to 4.5 years after a patient has been placed on therapy. Thus, the potential for any drug to present with an adverse idiosyncratic reaction at anytime must always be remembered.

One of the most common idiosyncratic reactions is the appearance of "drug rashes;" however, different types of idiosyncratic drug interactions can occur at different times in the same patient. We are all aware of the valproic acid idiosyncratic interactions which range from the undesirable but nonlife-threatening alopecia to fatal hepatotoxicity. These interactions are concisely summarized in the report of Dreifuss et al.

It is possible for a patient to experience multiple idiosyncratic reactions simultaneously or sequentially. The underlying mechanisms of each idiosyncratic reaction can be strikingly variable depending on the physiological or biochemical system involved in the reaction. Thus, the valproic acid-produced hyperammonemia, alopecia, and acute pancreatitis or hepatotoxicity are all idiosyncratic drug reactions each initiated by alterations of different physiological and/or biochemical systems. It is generally believed that the increased blood ammonia concentrations following valproate therapy are related to an alteration of carnitine catabolism, whereas the mechanisms for the development of acute pancreatitis or hepatotoxicity appear to be unrelated to elevated blood ammonia concentrations. Valproate-induced alopecia is probably related to a marginal zinc deficiency that occurs in some patients during valproate therapy.

For decades we have been searching for analytical techniques that would allow identification of those patients who are at risk to develop idiosyncratic drug reactions while receiving any drug therapy. Ideally, one would like to be in a position where a series of biochemical or physiological tests could establish whether or not a patient is at risk to develop an idiosyncratic reaction prior to the time they are placed on a specific therapeutic regimen. To date, the achievement of this goal has remained elusive because our understanding of the mechanisms which precipitate idiosyncratic reactions remains obscure. Clearly, we must continue to search for new and unique diagnostic techniques that will allow us to identify those patients who are at risk to develop idiosyncratic and/or drug–drug interactions.

DRUG–DRUG INTERACTIONS

These interactions occur with the concomitant administration of two or more drugs. The most common drug–drug interactions are associated with decreased clearance rates and increased plasma concentrations of the drug whose clearance is being inhibited as a consequence of the drug–drug interaction. The elevated drug concentrations are usually associated with a change in the patient's clinical status (e.g., the development of clinical signs of drug intoxication). (A classic example of a drug–drug interaction is the development of clinical phenytoin or carbamazepine drug intoxication following the administration of erythromycin or cimetidine.) Conversely, it is also possible that the simultaneous administration of multiple drugs may result in a decrease in total plasma drug concentrations rather than an increase. This phenomenon is usually associated with enhanced drug clearance rates that occur either by (1) a direct induction of microsomal enzymes responsible for a drug or (2) the displacement of a drug from its protein-binding site, which increases the free drug concentrations and causes an enhanced drug clearance. Decreased plasma drug concentrations ultimately lead to an exacerbation of the disease process and a loss of therapeutic control.

The distinguishing feature between these two enhanced drug-clearance interactions is the time-course required for the development of the interaction. If the decreased plasma drug concentration is secondary to the induction of microsomal drug-metabolizing enzymes, there is a gradual change in plasma drug concentrations of the drug whose clearance rate is being enhanced. Drug concentration changes are dependent upon the synthesis rate of additional microsomal (P-450) drug-metabolizing enzymes which takes place gradually over a period of weeks. When a drug induces its own metabolism, this phenomenon is commonly referred to as induction or as autoinduction. Autoinduction is more pronounced with some drugs than with others. Carbamazepine induces its own metabolism. Often within 1 week of carbamazepine therapy, plasma concentrations are optimal and usually seizure control is achieved in most patients. If the patient is maintained on the same dose (mg/kg) for 1 month, upon reanalysis, carbamazepine concentrations will be 40–50% lower than the original values. This decrease is secondary to the synthesis of additional carbamazepine-metabolizing enzymes within the microsomal P-450 drug-metabolizing system. Because more enzyme is now available to metabolize the drug, the carbamazepine clearance rate increases and the plasma and tissue concentrations fall. Clinically, the previously well-controlled patient may experience breakthrough seizures as the plasma concentrations become suboptimal. Multiple drug therapy, even with drugs which are not of the same class, can also induce drug-metabolizing enzyme concentrations and enhance drug clearance rates.

In contrast, if the drug interaction is the result of a drug's displacement from its protein-binding sites, the fall in the total plasma concentrations can be extremely rapid (within hours) as the displaced free drug is cleared. Under these circumstances, a new total and free steady-state drug concentration will be reached within five drug half-lives. The classic example of a protein-binding displacement interaction is observed following administration of valproic acid (VPA) to patients stabilized on phenytoin. VPA has greater affinity for the drug-binding sites on albumin than does phenytoin. VPA displaces phenytoin from its protein-binding sites, thus increasing the free plasma phenytoin concentrations. The displaced (free) phenytoin is now available to enter the hepatocyte where it is rapidly metabolized. Thus, the clearance rate of phenytoin is enhanced and a new equilibrium between total and free phenytoin is established at lower total drug concentrations. Clinically, it is quite common to encounter a 30–50% drop in a patient's total phenytoin concentration within 24 hours following the addition of VPA to the therapeutic regimen. VPA also displaces carbamazepine from its protein-binding sites with a resultant increase in free carbamazepine concentrations to levels that may precipitate clinical carbamazepine toxicity in the patient.

Clinically, drug–drug interactions of any type may be characterized by either a dramatic or subtle change in the patient's clinical status. If the plasma concentration of an antiepileptic drug has increased, the end result will usually be the development of clinical signs of drug toxicity. Conversely, if the antiepileptic drug concentration has decreased, one expects to see an exacerbation of seizures. Our clinical experience has taught us that when drugs, which inhibit drug metabolism or displace a drug from its protein-binding sites, are added to a patient's therapeutic regimen, clinical

Table 4-1. Phenytoin Drug Interactions

Drug	Effectiveness	PHT concentration	Mechanism
Allopurinol	Increased	Increased	Enzyme inhibition
Amiodarone	Increased	Increased	Unknown
Antacids	Reduced	Reduced	Reduced absorption or rapid
Anticoagulants			
Dicumarol	Increased	Increased	Complicated
Coumadin	Variable	Variable	Complicated
Antineoplastic agents	Decreased	Reduced	Unknown—reduced absorption
Phenobarbital	Increased	Increased	Complicated—dependent
	Decreased	Decreased	on enzyme induction
	No change	No change	state
Benzodiazepines	Increased	Increased	Enzyme inhibition
Carbamazepine	Increased	Increased	Complicated—dependent
	Decreased	Decreased	on enzyme induction
	No change	No change	state
Chloral hydrate	Decreased	Decreased	Unknown
Chloramphenicol	Increased	Increased	Enzyme inhibition
Chlorpheniramine	Increased	Increased	Unknown
Generic phenytoin	Variable	Variable	Variable absorption?
Cimetidine	Increased	Increased	Enzyme inhibition
Diazoxide	Decreased	Reduced	Enzyme induction
Disulfiram	Increased	Increased	Enzyme inhibition
Folic acid	Reduced	Reduced	Complicated—induction

signs of the drug–drug interaction are usually apparent within three to five half-lives of the drug whose clearance has been altered. Thus, patients who have erythromycin added to their carbamazepine therapy will begin to exhibit carbamazepine toxicity within 2 to 3 days following the institution of erythromycin therapy. In contrast, following the addition of a drug which induces drug metabolism, we would not expect to see the clinical signs of induction until 3 to 4 weeks following the institution of the new drug therapy. At that time the patient may experience breakthrough seizures.

In summary, drug–drug interactions are easily identified because there is usually a clear-cut clinical marker (the development of adverse side effects or an exacerbation of the disease process) that indicates that a drug–drug interaction is occurring. Therefore, many drug–drug interactions can be identified simply by carefully monitoring a patient's clinical status before and after any change in his therapeutic regimen. Quantitation of the patient's drug concentrations identifies which drugs are interacting.

Table 4-1. *(cont'd)*

Drug	Effectiveness	PHT concentration	Mechanism
Ibuprofen	Increased	Increased	Unknown inhibition
Isoniazid	Increased	Increased	Enzyme inhibition
Loxapine	Decreased	Reduced	Unknown
Methylphenidate	Increased	Increased	Inhibition dependent on
	No change	No change	drug metabolism states
Metronidazole	Increased	Increased	Enzyme inhibition
Miconazole	Increased	Increased	Enzyme inhibition
Nitrofurantoin	Decreased	Reduced	Enzyme induction
Phenacemide	Increased	Increased	Enzyme inhibition
Phenothiazines	Increased	Increased	Complicated—dependent
Chlorpromazine	Decreased		on induction
Thioridazine	No change		
Phenylbutazones	Increased	Increased	Enzyme inhibition protein-binding displacement
Propoxyphene	Increased	Increased	Enzyme inhibition
Pyridoxine	Decreased	Reduced	Unknown—enzyme induction
Rifampin	Decreased	Reduced	Enzyme induction
Salicylates	Increased	Increased	Protein-binding displacement
Succinimides	Increased	Increased	Enzyme inhibition
Sucralfate	Decreased	Reduced	Decreased absorption
Sulfonamides	Increased	Increased	Enzyme inhibition

Once a drug–drug interaction has been identified, appropriate alteration of the patient's therapeutic regimen will eliminate the interaction and the patient's clinical status will return to its previous level as the drug concentrations return to their previous values over a finite time interval. Ideally, one should be searching for ways to identify those drugs which are apt to precipitate drug–drug interactions prior to their addition to the patient's therapeutic regimen. Clearly, any drug whose chemical structure and properties assure that its protein binding, hepatic metabolic pathways, or renal excretion patterns are similar to those of the currently marketed antiepileptic drugs would have the potential to precipitate a drug–drug interaction.

Drug–drug interactions are most commonly encountered during adjunctive therapy when the patient is simultaneously receiving drug treatment for an acute illness or when chronic drug therapy is introduced to treat a highly developed disease. The following sections deal with antiepileptic drug–drug interactions although the principles are applicable to other drugs as well (Tables 4-1 to 4-6).

Table 4-2. Carbamazepine Drug Interactions

Drug	Effectiveness	CBZ concentration	Mechanism
Androgens	Increased	Increased	Enzyme inhibition
Phenobarbital	Reduced	Reduced	Complicated—dependent
	Increased	Increased	on enzyme induction
	No change	No change	state
Cimetidine	Increased	Increased	Enzyme inhibition
Danazol	Increased	Increased	Enzyme inhibition
Diltiazem	Increased	Increased	Enzyme inhibition
Erythromycin	Increased	Increased	Enzyme inhibition
Isoniazid	Increased	Increased	Enzyme inhibition
Nicotinamide	Increased	Increased	Enzyme inhibition
Propoxyphene	Increased	Increased	Enzyme inhibition
Troleandomycin	Increased	Increased	Enzyme inhibition
Verapamil	Increased	Increased	Enzyme inhibition
Generic carbamazepine	Variable	Variable	Variable absorption?

ABSORPTION OF ANTIEPILEPTIC DRUGS IS ALTERED BY OTHER DRUGS

It is well established that the concomitant administration of antacids with antiepileptic drugs (as well as other drugs) may significantly decrease drug absorption. Antacids contain high concentrations of calcium, magnesium, and aluminum salts. Coadministration of an antacid with an antiepileptic drug results in a chemical reaction whereby sodium salt or the

Table 4-3. Valproic Acid Drug Interactions

Drug	Effectiveness	VPA concentration	Mechanism
Antacids	Increased	Decreased	Decreased absorption
Carbamazepine	Increased	Increased	Complicated—dependent
	Decreased	Decreased	on enzyme induction
	No change	No change	state
Phenothiazines Chlorpromazine	Increased	Increased	Enzyme inhibition
Salicylates	Increased	Increased	Protein-binding displacement
			Enzyme inhibition
Generic valproic acid	Variable	Variable	Variable absorption?

Table 4-4. Primidone Drug Interactions

Drug	Effectiveness	PRM concentration	Mechanism
Carbamazepine	Increased	Increased	Enzyme induction
Carbonic anhydrase inhibitors and acetazolamide	Decreased	Decreased	Decreased absorption
Phenytoin	Increased	Increased	Complicated enzyme induction conversion to phenobarbital enhanced
	Decreased	Decreased	
Isoniazid	Increased	Increased	Enzyme inhibition decreased conversion to phenobarbital
Nicotinamide	Increased	Increased	Enzyme inhibition decreased conversion to phenobarbital
Generic primidone	Variable	Variable	Variable absorption?

free acid of an antiepileptic drug is converted into a calcium, magnesium, or aluminum salt that is significantly less soluble in water than the sodium salt. This decreased water solubility prevents the antiepileptic drug from entering the solution which is necessary for uptake by the absorption sites in the intestinal wall. Clinically, the decreased absorption of antiepileptic drugs during concomitant antacid administration is characterized by an exacerbation of seizures. This interaction between antacids and antiepileptic drugs can be easily prevented simply by administering the antacid at least 4 hours before or after the antiepileptic drug administration.

Table 4-5. Phenobarbital Drug Interactions

Drug	Effectiveness	PB concentration	Mechanism
Phenacemide	Increased	Increased	Enzyme inhibition
Propoxyphene	Increased	Increased	Enzyme inhibition
Pyridoxine	Reduced	Decreased	Unknown
Rifampin	Decreased	Decreased	Enzyme induction
Valproic acid	Increased	Increased	Complicated enzyme inhibition and change in urine pH to enhance phenobarbital reabsorption

Table 4-6. Drug Interactions in Which Other Drug Concentrations and Effects Are Altered by Antiepileptic Drugs

Antiepileptic drug	Drug affected		
	Increased plasma concentration/effect	Decreased plasma concentration/effect	
Phenytoin	Phenobarbital	Dexamethasone Dicumarol Digitoxin Doxycycline Lidocaine Nortriptyline Oral contraceptives	Pethidine Prednisolone Pyridoxine Theophylline Thyroxine Antipyrine	Clonazepam Haloperidol Salicylates Acetaminophen Cyclosporine
Phenobarbital	—	Chloramphenicol Cimetidine Documarol Digitoxin Doxycycline Dexamethasone	Griseofulvin Nortriptyline Phenylbutazone Warfarin Cyclosporine Metoprolol Propranolol	
Primidone	Phenytoin	See phenobarbital		
Carbamazepine	—	Doxycycline Warfarin Cyclosporine		

GENERIC ANTIEPILEPTIC DRUGS ARE A SPECIAL CONSIDERATION

The widespread practice of administering generic drugs as a means of decreasing patient cost has become widespread. The United States Food and Drug Administration has certified a wide variety of generic drugs as bioequivalent to the "brand name" product. It is to be emphasized that the administration of a specific chemical will produce the same pharmacological effect whether it is a generic or a brand name product. The problem is that different generic manufacturers often use different excipient lubricants, fillers, or manufacturing processes which can alter either the rate of dissolution or the bioavailability of the generic preparation. It is these differences in manufacturing processes which lead to the failure of generic drugs and not the drug contained in the preparation.

Following the introduction of various generic phenytoin preparations, some patients were observed to have periods of transient phenytoin toxicity whereas others had an exacerbation of seizures. The Food and Drug Administration reclassified phenytoin into two categories: that which was readily absorbed, the so-called "fast" phenytoin, and "slow" phenytoin, which was absorbed at a slower rate (Parke-Davis, Dilantin). The introduction of generic carbamazepine, primidone, and valproic acid have all been followed by numerous reports of an exacerbation of seizures or transient drug intoxication.

In contrast to many other therapeutic agents, the antiepileptic drugs have an extremely narrow therapeutic range. Thus, an increase in total plasma concentrations by 20% can lead to the development of adverse side effects, whereas a 20% decrease in concentration can lead to breakthrough seizures. Because of the narrow therapeutic range of the antiepileptic drugs, it is strongly recommended that patients placed on antiepileptic drug therapy be maintained on the same preparation throughout their course of therapy. The appropriate titration of plasma concentrations to the desired range in relation to the therapeutic goal should be carried out with each generic preparation. Clinicians face a major problem with respect to generic drugs because of the mandatory substitution laws and the pharmacist's option to substitute any generic preparation, regardless of manufacturer, without the necessity of notifying the physician that the patient's generic brand of antiepileptic drug has been changed. The end result is that patients, even on generic drugs, can exhibit wide fluctuations in their antiepileptic drug concentrations, and the clinical course which in reality is solely dependent upon which generic manufacturer made the drug. For this reason, we strongly urge that all patients treated with antiepileptic drugs be maintained on the same preparation by the same manufacturer.

Most major antiepileptic drugs for which a generic preparation is available has had one or more lots of drug recalled owing to failures in the manufacturing process which resulted in decreased bioavailability and patient breakthrough seizures or toxicity. For this reason, we emphasize that every clinician must discuss generic antiepileptic drugs with every patient in order to alert him about the hazards of randomly switching drug brands and to underscore the importance of prescriptions being dispensed as written whether they are for the brand name product or for a specific generic antiepileptic drug.

ANTIEPILEPTIC DRUGS CAN BE DISPLACED FROM THEIR PROTEIN-BINDING SITES

The protein binding of most drugs is low enough that even major changes in free drug concentration secondary to altered binding are not clinically significant in drug interactions. However, it is well established that for drugs which are more than 80–90% protein bound, changes in free drug concentration and therapeutic response can be precipitated by altering the protein-binding pattern of the drug (see Chapter 3). Of the antiepileptic drugs, only phenytoin (90%) and valproic acid (95%) readily participate in drug displacement reactions associated with protein binding. Valproic acid has a greater affinity for the albumin-binding sites than all of the other antiepileptic drugs; therefore it has the capacity to displace phenytoin as well as other drugs from their protein bindings. It is for this reason that patients receiving either carbamazepine or phenytoin can exhibit drug–drug interactions secondary to elevated free concentrations. In the case of phenytoin, the levels may be either increased or decreased (see Chapter 3). Valproic acid displaces carbamazepine from its protein-binding sites in such a manner that the free carbamazepine and carbamazepine-epoxide concentrates may be toxic even in the presence of normal total levels. Whenever a patient exhibits clinical signs of drug intoxication, which are not associated with marked alterations of total levels, free drug concentrations should be determined to assess whether the toxicity is from drug interactions that may have increased the free drug concentrations.

ANTIEPILEPTIC DRUGS INDUCE THEIR OWN METABOLISM

Because all drugs are recognized as toxic foreign compounds by the body, it follows that the presence of a drug stimulates the organism to eliminate the toxin. Hepatic drug metabolism is routinely carried out within the microsomal fraction by several cytochrome P-450 isoenzymes. It is known that these enzymes are also responsible for steroid metabolism. Therefore sufficient concentrations of drug-metabolizing enzymes are always present to metabolize small quantities (i.e., a single or a few repeated doses) at all times. When drugs are administered chronically, the available P-450 enzymes have insufficient capacity to metabolize the drug load. Therefore, the feedback mechanisms present in hepatocytes call down the synthesis of more P-450 isoenzymes to metabolize the additional drug. The synthesis of more drug-metabolizing enzymes is commonly referred to as enzyme induction.

There are two key points which must always be considered with respect to enzyme induction. (1) The P-450 isoenzymes responsible for drug metabolism are capable of interacting with many classes of drugs. For example, the hydroxylation of phenytoin, phenobarbital, nirvanol, acetaminophen, acetylsalicylic acid (aspirin), and many other aromatic compounds are carried out by the same P-450 isoenzyme. (2) There is a maximum limit to the absolute concentration of P-450 isoenzymes that can be synthesized. Therefore, if a patient is already maximally induced, the addition of another drug which is metabolized by the same pathway (i.e., by the same isoenzyme), will not result in a significant further induction of drug metabolism.

CARBAMAZEPINE AUTOINDUCTION IS A SPECIAL CASE

It is well established that following chronic therapy, carbamazepine induces its own metabolism through a stimulation of the hepatic microsomal drug-metabolizing enzyme systems. Studies in both adults and children have demonstrated that following 30 days of therapy, there is an increased carbamazepine clearance rate, a decreased carbamazepine half-life, and an average decrease of serum steady-state carbamazepine concentrations by as much as 40–50%. It is to be noted that following the initial autoinduction period of 3–6 weeks, there is no further significant increase in carbamazepine clearance rates during continued therapy. This stabilization of carbamazepine clearance rates suggests that the hepatic synthesis of drug-metabolizing enzymes responsible for metabolism reaches a maximum rate of activity. Once the maximum rate is reached, further induction does not occur.

The autoinduction of carbamazepine has major clinical significance. A patient initially starting on carbamazepine therapy will achieve therapeutic serum concentrations within 5–6 days. However, as the autoinduction process proceeds, the carbamazepine serum concentrations will decrease to suboptimal concentrations and seizure activity can reappear. Therefore, it is advisable that serum concentrations of carbamazepine be reevaluated 4–6 weeks following the initiation of therapy. Appropriate adjustments in the patient's dosage regimen should be made to optimize the serum concentrations and the drug concentrations monitored 2 weeks later to insure achievement of the desired concentration. Again it is emphasized that hepatic drug metabolism rates are also influenced by both genetic factors and the presence of concomitant drug therapy. Therefore, the degree of autoinduction in a given patient following the initiation of carbamazepine therapy can exhibit wide variability. Dosage adjustments should not be made without monitoring the patient's drug concentration and current clinical status. These principles apply not only to the clinical management of the epilepsies but also the clinical management of manic depression (see Chapter 7).

ANTIEPILEPTIC DRUGS INDUCE THE METABOLISM OF OTHER DRUGS

Antiepileptic drugs have the ability to induce their own metabolism and induce the metabolism of concomitantly administered drugs as well. Addition of antiepileptic drugs into the therapeutic regimen of patients already receiving other chronic drug therapy may result in an enhanced clearance rate, decreased half-lives, and decreased steady-state serum concentrations of the original agents. Drugs whose metabolism has been reported to be induced by antiepileptic drugs are listed in Table 4-6.

OTHER DRUGS INDUCE THE METABOLISM OF ANTIEPILEPTIC DRUGS

As indicated above and in Chapter 3, many drugs have the capacity to induce the hepatic drug metabolism of P-450 isoenzyme systems. Thus, patients who have been stabilized on a specific antiepileptic dosage may exhibit enhanced antiepileptic clearance, a decreased half-life, and decreased serum drug concentrations following the addition of another drug to the patient's therapeutic regimen (see Tables 4-1 to 4-6). In addition, the enhanced metabolism of carbamazepine by other drugs results in increased serum concentrations of carbamazepine 10,11-epoxide (the major metabolite of carbamazepine). Recent evidence suggests that elevated carbamazepine-epoxide concentrations are related to the development of carbamazepine clinical toxicity.

Clinically it must always be remembered that a wide variety of drugs have the capacity to enhance hepatic clearance of other drugs. Therefore, whenever a patient is receiving polytherapy or another drug is added to a monotherapy regimen, the potential for drug–drug interactions is high. Under these circumstances, following a change in a patient's therapeutic regimen, drug concentrations should be routinely monitored and appropriate changes made in the patient's therapeutic regimen based upon the patient's clinical status, serum concentrations, and desired therapeutic goals.

Interpatient variability of the mechanisms regulating drug-enzyme induction are common. Clearly, polytherapy can significantly alter antiepileptic clearance and vice versa. Monitoring drug concentrations is an efficient means of adjusting for the individual variability in these responses.

OTHER DRUGS INHIBIT THE METABOLISM OF CARBAMAZEPINE

The hepatic microsomal drug-metabolizing enzyme systems responsible for antiepileptic metabolism can be readily inhibited. Inhibition of drug metabolism and consequent drug toxicity has greater clinical implications than does enzyme induction. Generally, inhibition of drug metabolism is competitive and reversible when the inhibiting agent is removed. The onset of clinical signs of drug intoxication following enzyme inhibition is rapid. Drug clearance is decreased, drug half-lives are prolonged, and steady-state serum drug concentrations are elevated following enzyme inhibition. These changes begin immediately upon addition of the inhibiting drug to a patient's therapeutic regimen. Serum concentrations will reach their maximum levels at seven half-lives after introduction of the inhibiting agent. However, clinical symptoms of drug intoxication will appear as soon as the serum concentrations exceed the minimum toxic concentration even though a new steady state has not been reached.

The severity of a drug–drug interaction secondary to enzyme inhibition is dependent upon two factors: (1) In competitive inhibition, the amount of enzyme inhibited is dependent upon the concentration of the inhibiting agent. Inhibition-related drug–drug interactions have been reported in some patients yet their existence has not been confirmed by other investigators. Retrospective analysis often demonstrates that those patients who exhibited the drug interaction received higher doses of the inhibiting agents than those patients who did not exhibit the interaction. (2) Chronic exposure to an inhibiting agent has a greater probability of producing a drug–drug interaction than does intermittent exposure to the same agent. The reason for this difference is that patients receiving intermittent doses of an inhibitor partially clear the inhibitor drug thus releasing an enzyme that had previously been inhibited, thus a new steady state is not achieved. In contrast, chronic drug therapy provides a constant inhibition of the drug-metabolizing enzymes, thus allowing the concentrations of the drug whose metabolism has been inhibited to increase to a new steady-state concentration which is often above the minimal toxic concentration and thus precipitates adverse side effects in the patient. The compounds listed in Tables 4-1 to 4-6 have been reported to produce clinical toxicity of antiepileptic drugs through their ability to competitively inhibit the cytochrome P-450 hepatic drug-metabolizing system, reduce drug clearance, and elevate serum drug concentrations.

CLINICAL PERSPECTIVE OF ANTIEPILEPTIC DRUG INTERACTIONS

The most commonly encountered drug–drug interactions associated with antiepileptic therapy occur in epileptic patients who became acutely ill, for example, children or adults placed on macrolide antibiotic therapy for infection control. (Erythromycin or troleandomycin are potent competitive inhibitors of the hepatic microsomal drug-enzyme systems.) Usually the patient is seen for the acute infective illness by a primary care physician who prescribes a 10-day course of antibiotic therapy without considering the potential for a drug–drug interaction. After 3–5 days of antibiotic therapy, the patient develops the classic symptoms of antiepileptic drug intoxication, nystagmus, diplopia, nausea, vomiting ataxia, and lethargy. Measurement of serum antiepileptic drug levels yields values ranging above the minimum toxic concentrations. This toxicity is readily reversible by discontinuing antiepileptic drug therapy until serum concentrations reach optimal levels and then reinstating the antiepileptic drug at a lower dose. A better solution, if possible, is to discontinue macrolide antibiotic therapy and substitute a different antibiotic drug. The same drug interaction also commonly occurs in postsurgical patients who have been placed on prophylactic macrolide antibiotic therapy.

It is essential to remember that following the completion of the antibiotic course, the antiepileptic clearance rate will again increase to its previous levels. Therefore, if the dose had been reduced during macrolide antibiotic therapy, it must be increased in steps to its previous level. Again it is advantageous to monitor the antiepileptic drug concentrations immediately prior to reinstating therapy and 5–7 days (steady state) after the final dosage increment.

In contrast to those drugs which are prescribed for relatively short intervals, there exists a group of drugs in which prolonged therapy is necessary. Cimetidine is a potent competitive enzyme inhibitor commonly prescribed for long intervals. Patients receiving antiepileptic therapy who are placed on a cimetidine regimen for ulcer control should have their antiepileptic drug therapy reduced appropriately (in our experience the deletion of one dose per day is usually sufficient) immediately upon initiation of cimetidine. Serum drug concentrations should be monitored within 1 week of the therapy change and final adjustments made.

It is equally important to promptly readjust the patient's antiepileptic regimen immediately upon the discontinuation of cimetidine therapy. Failure to adjust the antiepileptic drug regimen will result in decreased serum concentrations within 5–7 days. Thus, the patient is at a higher risk to have breakthrough seizures. We note that ranitidine is not a significant inhibitor of hepatic drug metabolism. Therefore, it would appear to be a more appropriate first-choice drug when an H2-antagonist is required in patients receiving antiepileptic or other drug therapy.

Propoxyphene is also a competitive inhibitor of the hepatic drug-metabolism enzyme system. Usually, elevation of antiepileptic drug concentrations occurs following the postsurgical administration of propoxyphene for pain control or during chronic propoxyphene administration. Generally, the intermittent use of propoxyphene does not cause the development of clinical toxicity because the propoxyphene concentrations are not sufficiently high enough over a prolonged interval to inhibit antiepileptic drug clearance. Thus, even though a slight elevation in steady-state antiepileptic drug concentrations can occur, the inhibition may be insufficient to produce a clinical toxicity.

Isoniazid is another competitive inhibitor of antiepileptic drug metabolism. Because this drug is administered chronically, it is essential that the patient's antiepileptic regimen be adjusted with the initiation of isoniazid therapy and again upon the discontinuation of isoniazid therapy.

In summary, any patient who receives multiple drug therapy is at risk of developing a drug–drug interaction. Those drugs which induce the hepatic microsomal system cause enhanced drug clearance, decreased half-lives, and decreased serum concentrations. The changes in drug clearance develop slowly, usually over a period of several weeks. Patients are at risk for an exacerbation of seizures as the antiepileptic drug concentrations fall to suboptimal concentrations. Drugs which inhibit the hepatic microsomal enzyme systems cause decreased drug clearance, prolonged half-lives, and elevated serum concentrations. The changes in drug clearance following enzyme inhibition develop rapidly, usually within days. As the serum drug concentrations cross the minimum toxic concentration, the patient usually develops the clinical signs and symptoms of drug intoxication. Drug–drug interactions are preventable. It is the responsibility of every physician to be alert for potential drug interactions whenever a change in the patient's therapeutic regimen is initiated. The clinical management of the epilepsies requires careful administration of a variety of drugs. There is nothing more frustrating than watching a previously well-controlled patient experience an exacerbation of seizures or develop a drug toxicity which could have been prevented simply by an appropriate adjustment of the patient's therapeutic regimen. Such events are often a direct consequence of a failure in communication between the neurologist or psychiatrist and the primary care physician. It is our responsibility to educate our colleagues to potential drug–drug interactions and to insure that the communication between the primary care physician and the specialist is active rather than passive and prospective rather than retrospective. Such an effort will lead to the prevention of drug–drug interactions thus insuring a better quality of life for our patients.

SUGGESTED READING

Bertilsson L, Hojer B, Tybring G, Osterloh J, Rane A. Autoinduction of carbamazepine metabolism in children examined by a stable isotope technique. *Clin Pharmacol Ther* 1980;27:83–88.

Bowdle TA, Levy RH, Cutler RE. Effects of carbamazepine on valproic acid in normal man. *Clin Pharmacol Ther* 1979;26:629–634.

Carranco E, Kareus J, Co S, Peak V, Al-Rajeh S. Carbamazepine toxicity induced by concurrent erythromycin therapy. *Arch Neurol* 1985;42:187–188.

Christiansen J, Dam M. Drug interaction in epileptic patients. In: Schneider H, Janz D, Gardner-Thorp C, Meinardi H, Sherwin AL, eds. *Clinical Pharmacology of Anti-Epileptic Drugs.* Berlin: Springer-Verlag, 1975:197–200.

Dravet C, Mesdjian E, Cenraud B, Roger J. Interaction between carbamazepine and triacetyloleandomycin. *Lancet* 1977;1:810–811.

Gilman AG, Goodman LS, Rall TW, Murad F. *The Pharmacological Basis of Therapeutics,* 7th ed. New York: Macmillan, 1985.

Morselli PL, Pippenger CE, Penry JK, eds. *Antiepileptic Drug Therapy in Pediatrics.* New York: Raven Press, 1983.

Pellock, JM. Carbamazepine side effects in adults and children. *Epilepsia (Suppl. 3)* 1987;564–570.

Pippenger CE. *Therapeutic Drug Monitoring: Pharmacologic Principles, Diagnostic Medicine.* Oradell, NJ: Medical Economics Company, Inc., 1983.

Schmidt D. *Adverse Effects of Antiepileptic Drugs.* New York: Raven Press, 1982.

Webster LK, Mihaly GW, Jones DB, Smallwood RA, Phillips JA, Vajda FJ. Effect of cimetidine and ranitidine on carbamazepine and sodium valproate pharmacokinetics. *Eur J Clin Pharmacol* 1984;27:341–343.

Wong YY, Ludden TM, Bell RD. Effect of erythromycin on carbamazepine kinetics. *Clin Pharmacol Ther* 1983;33:460–464.

Woodbury DM, Penry JK, Pippenger CE, eds. *Antiepileptic Drugs,* 2nd ed. New York: Raven Press, 1982.

5

Pharmacodynamics of Antiepileptic Drugs

C. E. Pippenger

The fundamental tenent of therapeutics and pharmacology is that all drugs have multiple actions at any given plasma concentration. It is well established that at a given plasma drug concentration, any drug has the capacity to interact with and alter the dynamics of more than one physiological system (see Chapter 3). The purpose of this chapter is to provide an overview of the mechanisms of action of antiepileptic drugs.

HISTORICAL BACKGROUND

Since antiquity, a wide variety of agents have been utilized to treat seizure disorders. The most commonly prescribed medications in medieval times were various herbal preparations and simple inorganic compounds. By the mid-nineteenth century, various inorganic salts of iron, iodine, zinc, copper, magnesium, and silver had been utilized for the treatment of epilepsy. Other commonly prescribed drugs included opium, digitalis, belladonna, mistletoe, and oil of wintergreen. None of these agents was particularly effective in controlling seizure disorders, although at toxic concentrations, all have the ability to depress the central nervous system.

Potassium bromide, introduced in 1857 for the treatment of epilepsy by Sir Charles Locok (Queen Victoria's obstetrician), was the first effective antiepileptic drug. At that time it was believed that epileptic seizures were caused by masturbation and bromide was recognized as a suppressant of libido. Following Locok's initial description, the prescription of bromide salts for the control of epilepsy increased significantly so that by the end of the 1800s, the National Hospital in London dispensed 2½ tons of bromides annually for the treatment of seizure disorders. It is interesting to note that the therapeutic index of bromides is extremely narrow and one of the most common clinical presentations of bromide toxicity is psychotic behavior. Prior to the introduction of bromides, epilepsy was reasonably tolerated by society. The introduction of bromides and the resultant increase in psychotic behavior among epileptics changed the attitude of society to the point where the epileptics were feared and shunned by their peers.

It was not until 1912 that the next antiepileptic drug, phenobarbital, was discovered. Its efficacy as an anticonvulsant was based upon the observation that when administered as a sedative to patients with a wide variety of seizure disorders, the seizure frequency decreased. Phenobarbital became the anticonvulsant drug of choice because it did not produce the adverse psychotic side effects commonly associated with bromides. It was not until 1937 that phenytoin, the first nonsedative antiepileptic drug, was described by Merritt and Putnam. Following the introduction of phenytoin, a number of structural and chemical analogues of the hydantoins were synthesized and marketed as anticonvulsants. Most of these analogues were less effective and had more adverse side effects than phenytoin. The more recent introduction of carbamazepine and valproic acid as major antiepileptic drugs represents the development of drugs which have fewer adverse side effects and are more effective in the treatment of seizure disorders.

Although at the present time, 18 drugs have been approved for use in the management of seizure disorders by the Food and Drug Administration in the United States, only 6 are used extensively. The major antiepileptic drugs are phenytoin, carbamazepine, phenobarbital, primidone, valproate, and ethosuximide. The other antiepileptic drugs, because of their potential to produce severe toxicity and their marginal effectiveness in most patients, should be utilized only in complex clinical situations by epileptologists. The use of these agents by general clinicians is not recommended.

MECHANISM OF ACTION

Historically, it was believed that in order for any compound to have antiepileptic activity, it was essential that the compound be a cyclic ureide (i.e., a primary ring structure that contains a combination of carbonyl and nitrogen groups). However, it is now established that this concept was incorrect because the most recently introduced and more effective antiepileptic drugs, carbamazepine and valproic acid, are not cyclic ureides. Currently, it is believed that a wide variety of different chemical structures have potential as antiepileptic agents.

All of the major antiepileptic drugs are considered to be membrane stabilizers (i.e., the regulation of seizure activity is achieved by either controlling the spread of the electrical activity which generates a clinical seizure from its focus or actually suppressing the focus itself). Thus, the major mechanism of action of carbamazepine, valproic acid, phenytoin, and primidone is the modification of ionic conductances across neuronal membranes. These drugs affect both sodium and calcium flux across excitable membranes. Consequently, the major antiepileptic drugs limit the high frequency-sustained neuronal discharges that generate in an epileptic focus from spreading to other cells. For example, it has been demonstrated that both carbamazepine and phenytoin can pass through a neuronal membrane and bind to a specific site located near the sodium channel on the internal surface of the membrane. Binding to this site delays reactivation of the sodium channel so that the cell cannot fire at a rapid rate.

It is to be noted that not all antiepileptic drugs work in exactly the same manner. For example, the barbiturates prolong γ-aminobutyric acid (GABA)-mediated synaptic inhibition by causing the chloride channel to remain open for longer periods of time. The prolonged opening of the chloride channel depresses neuronal activity. Benzodiazepines also depress neuronal activity through an alteration of chloride-channel response, however utilizing a different mechanism than that of phenobarbital. The benzodiazepines bind with a specific "benzodiazepine" receptor which regulates the GABA receptor and the benzodiazepine receptor stimulates the chloride channels to open more frequently after GABA stimulation. Valproic acid has the ability to limit high frequency-sustained neuronal discharges but also depresses neuronal activity by other mechanisms that remain to be elucidated.

An understanding of the pharmacodynamic mechanisms of action of antiepileptic drugs is important in selecting an appropriate drug for a particular seizure type. Antiepileptic drugs, on the basis of their mechanisms of action, can be divided into two types, specific and nonspecific. The specific antiepileptic drugs include carbamazepine, valproic acid, phenytoin, and primidone, each of which has the capacity to interfere with some aspect of seizure discharge and/or its spread. The nonspecific antiepileptic drugs (barbiturates and benzodiazepines) achieve seizure control by exerting a general depressant effect upon the central nervous system.

Based upon their mechanisms of action, the most appropriate drugs for various seizure types are summarized in Table 5-1. Most neurologists advocate the use of carbamazepine or phenytoin in the management of secondary generalized seizures and valproic acid for primary generalized seizures. It is without question to be emphasized that there is some overlap in the indications for usage of the major antiepileptic drugs. For example, both carbamazepine and phenytoin are effective in primary generalized seizures and there is strong evidence that valproate is effective in secondary generalized seizures. Without question, carbamazepine, phenytoin, and valproate are the three drugs of choice in the management of generalized convulsive seizure disorders. The other agents listed in Table 5-1 are uti-

Table 5-1. Effective Antiepileptic Drugs

Seizure type	Effective drug
Generalized convulsive	Phenytoin
	Carbamazepine
	Valproate
	Phenobarbital
	Primidone
	Clonazepam
	Clorazepate
	Acetazolamide
Generalized nonconvulsive absence	Valproate
	Ethosuximide
	Clonazepam
	Methsuximide
	(Phenobarbital)
Partial simple or complex	Carbamazepine
	Phenytoin
	Primidone
	Phenobarbital
	Valproate
	Clorazepate
	Methsuximide
	Clonozepam
	Acetazolamide

lized only as second-line drugs because they have unacceptable toxicities or are less effective antiepileptic agents.

The drugs of choice for the management of generalized nonconvulsive seizures, particularly absence seizures, are valproate and ethosuximide. Valproate is indicated for patients with absence seizures in combination with either myoclonic seizures or generalized tonic-clonic convulsions. In contrast, ethosuximide is the most effective primary agent in patients who have pure petit mal absence seizures with no other seizure types. Although clonazepam has been reported to be effective in generalized nonconvulsive seizures, its use is limited by its excessive sedative properties and the development of tolerance to its anticonvulsant effects in some patients. We emphasize that phenobarbital is absolutely ineffective in the management of absence seizures and of questionable value in mixed, generalized, nonconvulsive, seizure disorders. Clearly the drugs of choice for the treatment of simple partial or complex partial seizures are carbamazepine and phenytoin. Of the two, the lack of an impaired cognitive function by carbamazepine makes it the first drug of choice in the treatment of partial seizure disorders. It is noteworthy that valproate has been demonstrated to be clinically useful in conjunction with carbamazepine in those patients who do not respond to carbamazepine monotherapy.

Evaluation of the research data related to the pharmacodynamic mechanisms of the various antiepileptic drugs supports the concept that each antiepileptic drug's mechanism of action can be explained by the interaction of the drug with neuronal membranes to change the basic properties of the membranes, neurotransmitter synthesis and release, and/or alteration of other cellular metabolic processes. Therefore, for all of the major antiepileptic drugs, it appears probable that there is no single mechanism of action of that drug which can explain all of its pharmacodynamic effects. Although it is possible that there is one basic mechanism of effect on neuronal membranes which may result in antiepileptic drug activity, such a mechanism has yet to be elucidated.

Phenytoin

The major neuronal action of phenytoin is its ability to alter either passive or active transport mechanisms to regulate the flux of sodium and calcium across neuronal membranes. Intracellularly, the net effect in neuronal tissues appears to be a decrease in sodium influx which causes a decrease in intracellular sodium and calcium concentrations. The net effect of these ionic changes is a blockade of neurotransmitter release. It is to be emphasized, however, that at high tissue concentrations and in certain synapses, phenytoin may block the intracellular uptake of calcium by subcellular particles. This blockade of calcium uptake increases intracellular calcium concentrations and could cause increased transmitter release. This is why at high plasma concentrations, phenytoin actually can precipitate seizure activity. We emphasize that at plasma phenytoin concentrations above 35 μg/ml, patients may exhibit an exacerbation of seizures which is secondary to the excitatory effects of phenytoin. These seizures can be controlled simply by decreasing the phenytoin concentrations.

Carbamazepine

Not only does carbamazepine bind to type II Na^+ channels and inhibit influx, but it may affect calcium influx indirectly by its actions on adenosine receptors, peripheral-type benzodiazepine receptors, and $GABA_B$ (baclofen-like) activity. Anticonvulsant effects of carbamazepine on amygdala-kindled seizures have been most closely associated with effects at the peripheral-type benzodiazepine receptor and unblocked α_2-adrenergic receptors are required as yohimbine will reverse the anticonvulsant effects of carbamazepine.

Carbamazepine also exerts a panoply of acute and chronic effects on other neurotransmitter, neuromodulator, and peptide systems. Acutely, it decreases turnover of norepinephrine, dopamine, and GABA. It inhibits firing of the noradrenergic locus coeruleus neurons, while blocking norepinephrine release. Although it is structurally similar to the tricyclic antidepressant imipramine, its effects in blocking norepinephrine reuptake are not clinically relevant. Carbamazepine increases striatal acetylcholine and blocks adenylate cyclase activity stimulated by norepinephrine, adenosine, and ouabain. It also binds a platelet vasopressin receptor. Chronically, it decreases GABA turnover (more than acutely) and increases striatal substance P levels (an effect paralleled by lithium). Chronic administration also upregulates adenosine receptors in animals and peripheral-type benzodiazepine receptors in man. It also increases plasma tryptophan and decreases cerebrospinal fluid somatostatin. Chronic administration also affects dopamine and serotonin function, probably at a presynaptic level.

Although its anticonvulsant effects develop rapidly, the antidepressant effects of carbamazepine require 3–4 weeks to develop. This supports the concept that the underlying mechanism for carbamazepine's antiepileptic activity is different from its antidepressant mechanism. It also suggests that the psychotropic effects of carbamazepine are more likely related to chronic rather than acute effects of the drug.

Valproic Acid

The mechanism of action of valproic acid remains unclear. During the drug's initial introduction, there were a number of papers published supporting the concept of a valproic acid-induced increase in brain GABA concentrations. It was later established that the elevation of brain GABA levels in experimental models was achieved by valproic acid concentrations well above those encountered in a clinical situation. However, it is well recognized that valproate is a membrane stabilizer.

Clinical experience suggests that valproic acid exerts its effects through two different mechanisms. The immediate anticonvulsant effects of valproic acid observed over the first few days are probably attributable to its ability to produce acidosis on cerebral tissues (acidosis is an anticonvulsant and raises seizure thresholds, alkalosis is a convulsant and lowers seizure thresholds). The studies of Rowan et al. support the concept of a late onset and a persistent anticonvulsant effect for valproate. While monitoring via EEG the photoconvulsive response (PCR) in a group of epileptic patients, these investigators demonstrated that complete abolishment of the PCR-associated electrical activity required 3–4 weeks of valproate therapy. Conversely, when valproate therapy was discontinued in these patients, it was 3–4 weeks before the PCR activity, as recorded by EEG, returned to its previous levels even though the plasma valproate levels were undetectable within 72 hours. These and other studies support the concept of a long-term change in seizure threshold following valproate therapy. Based upon the chemical structure of valproic acid, it is interesting to speculate that valproate is actually incorporated into neuronal phospholipid membranes and "plugs leaks" in the membrane thus stabilizing the neuronal membrane. The turnover of phospholipid in the brain approximates the return of seizure activity in Rowan's absence study. This hypothetical mechanism has yet to be confirmed by the appropriate experiments.

Phenobarbital

The mechanism of action of phenobarbital remains unclear. It has been suggested that phenobarbital is uncharged at the acidic pH of brain epileptic foci; thus it is able to bind to the neuronal membrane within the focus to produce its antiepileptic effect. Phenobarbital has also been reported to enhance GABAergic inhibition, thus it more clearly may alter ionic conductance. Further studies are necessary to elucidate phenobarbital's anticonvulsant mechanisms.

Primidone

Although primidone is structurally similar to phenobarbital, its pharmacodynamic effects more closely resemble those of phenytoin and carbamazepine than those of phenobarbital. On the basis of the similarities of carbamazepine, phenytoin, and primidone in experimental models of epilepsy, it is hypothesized that primidone would affect sodium and calcium flux in a manner similar to phenytoin and carbamazepine. This concept is supported by the clinical observation that primidone, like phenytoin and carbamazepine, is effective in the control of complex partial seizures, whereas phenobarbital is absolutely ineffective in controlling complex partial seizures.

Ethosuximide

The mechanism of action of ethosuximide remains to be elucidated. To date there is no direct evidence linking ethosuximide to central nervous system (CNS) neurotransmitters. It is hypothesized that ethosuximide may alter receptor responses to inhibitory neurotransmitters although the evidence is far from convincing. Based on the clinical and electrophysiological characteristics of absence seizures, one can speculate that the physiological or biochemical system responsible for the generation of absence seizures is not severe, therefore subtle changes in the ionic flux of sodium or calcium across neuronal membranes may be sufficient to control the abnormal neuronal activity associated with absence seizures. We would anticipate that ethosuximide may stabilize ionic flux within the absence focus.

DRUGS EFFECTIVE IN PSYCHIATRIC DISEASE

A detailed description of mechanisms of action of those drugs utilized in the management of various psychiatric diseases is beyond the scope of this chapter. However, the fact that any drug which affects neuronal activity, whether as an antiepileptic or an antipsychotic drug, would be anticipated to have some effect on the clinical manifestations of any disease process within the central nervous system. These drug classes do have certain similarities. It is particularly noteworthy that the anticonvulsant drug carbamazepine has found widespread application in the medical management of bipolar and depressive illness (see Chapter 7). It is also extensively utilized in certain types of pain (trigeminal neuralgia). Clearly the ability of carbamazepine to alter neuronal functions to regulate seizures, and the ability of carbamazepine to regulate the physiological and biochemical changes associated with depression, demonstrate that the versatility of these compounds possess similar mechanisms in controlling neurological disease.

Historically the tricyclic antidepressants were believed to alleviate the disease process by their ability to block the reuptake of norepinephrine and serotonin at the presynaptic monoaminergic neuron. Recent studies of the neuropharmacological effects of the antidepressant drugs iprindole and mianserin have challenged this theory because neither of these drugs significantly blocks the reuptake of either norepinephrine or serotonin. One of the physiological theories to explain depression, commonly referred to as the dysregulation hypothesis, states that there is a failure in the regulating mechanisms controlling the neurotransmitter systems which results in an imbalance of neurotransmitters at the receptor sites. Correction of the underlying depression precipitated by dysregulation would depend upon a rebalancing of the pre- and postsynaptic neurotransmitter concentrations within the noradrenergic system. It has been demonstrated that antidepressant therapy changes the sensitivity of various amine receptor systems. For example, long-term antidepressant therapy reduces the sensitivity of both postsynaptic β-adrenergic and the serotonin Type 2 receptors located on the postsynaptic membrane. It appears that the effect of antidepressant drugs on the presynaptic α_2-adrenergic receptors and the serotonin Type 1 receptor is negligible.

The use of lithium in controlling the manic episodes in bipolar disorders is well established (see Chapter 7). Experimental studies have demonstrated that lithium affects the synthesis, storage, release, or reuptake of norepinephrine, serotonin, dopamine, acetylcholine, and GABA. Lithium increases norepinephrine turnover but does not alter norepinephrine synthesis rates. Following chronic lithium administration, there is an increased uptake of norepinephrine but insignificant changes in norepinephrine turnover rates. Studies of adrenergic receptor sensitivity have yielded conflicting results. Lithium has been reported to reduce dopamine synthesis, increase dopamine turnover, and block dopamine sensitivity. It has been suggested that many of the neuronal membrane-stabilizing properties of lithium mimic those of known calcium channel-blocking agents. This may explain lithium's therapeutic efficacy in mania.

Because different disease processes are ultimately dependent upon the alteration of different physiological or biochemical systems, it follows that diseases which affect the central nervous system by whatever underlying physiological or biochemical abnormality will ultimately alter neuronal transmission and integration. It follows that the drugs utilized in the treatment of various psychiatric disorders, particularly bipolar illness and depression, may have their symptoms ameliorated by antiepileptic drugs which stabilize neuronal membranes. It is also worth noting that antiepileptic drugs and antidepressant drugs are typically not effective in regulating other types of psychiatric disease, perhaps with the exception of panic disorder. Therefore, the fundamental physiological and biochemical alterations in psychiatric disease which are not responsive to these agents must be elicited by different mechanisms.

In summary, the mechanism of action of drugs utilized in clinical management of various disease processes is only now being elucidated. Clearly, any drug which alters the fundamental physiological processes regulating neuronal activity at the ionic level should be effective in any disease process that alters neuronal activity at that level. The effectiveness of both antiepileptic drugs and antidepressant drugs in the treatment of bipolar and/or depressive illnesses support such a concept. An understanding of the mechanisms of action will lead to an understanding of the respective disease processes.

SUGGESTED READING

Delgado-Escueta AV, Ward AA, Jr, Woodbury DM, Porter RJ. *Basic Mechanisms of the Epilepsies.* New York: Raven Press, 1986.

Glaser GH, Penry JK, Woodbury DM. *Antiepileptic Drugs: Mechanisms of Action.* New York: Raven Press, 1980.

Rowan AJ, Binnie CD, Warfield, CA, Meinardi H, Meijer JWA. The delayed effect of sodium valproate on the photoconvulsive response in man. *Epilepsia* 1979;20:61–68.

Woodbury DM, Penry JK, Pippenger CE. *Antiepileptic Drugs,* 2nd ed. New York: Raven Press, 1982.

6

Behavioral Disorders in Childhood

Michael R. Trimble

As with adult psychiatry, classification in child psychiatry has been sub-ject to shifting boundaries. In this chapter, the diagnostic schema recom-mended in DSM IIIR is used, and the use of anticonvulsant drugs in certain childhood disorders is considered. The role of anticonvulsant drugs in mood disorders or schizophrenia-like conditions of children are not discussed, most of the relevant work which has been carried out being related to disruptive behavior and anxiety disorders.

DISRUPTIVE BEHAVIOR DISORDERS

DSM IIIR classifies these disorders as those that are socially disruptive, the behavior being more distressing to others than to people with the disorder. The main subclassifications are divided into attention-deficit hy-peractivity disorder (ADHD), conduct disorder, and oppositional-defiant disorder. The literature on anticonvulsants relates mainly to the first two subclassifications.

Attention-Deficit Hyperactivity Disorder

The development of the concept of ADHD has been intertwined with that of minimal cerebral dysfunction. Reports of severe behavior conse-quences of brain dysfunction in childhood stem from the early part of this century when hyperactivity and antisocial behavior were seen follow-ing encephalitis and head injury. Kahn and Cohen (1934) used the term "organic drivenness" to describe such behavior patterns, the assumption being that these behaviors were a sequelae of organic brain damage, albeit often subtle.

Laufer et al. (1956) described the hyperkinetic impulse disorder, the main features being hyperactivity, short attention span, impulsivity, irritability, poor frustration tolerance, poor school work, and visuomotor difficulties. DSM II had the category "hyperkinetic reaction of childhood," DSM III using the term "attention-deficit disorder." The diagnostic criteria for ADHD from DSM IIIR are shown in Table 6-1. The spectrum

Table 6-1. Diagnostic Criteria for 314.01 Attention-Deficit Hyperactivity Disorder (ADHD)

Note: Consider a criterion met only if the behavior is considerably more frequent than that of most people of the same mental age

A. A disturbance of at least 6 months during which at least eight of the following are present:
1. Often fidgets with hands or feet or squirms in seat (in adolescents, may be limited to subjective feelings of restlessness)
2. Has difficulty remaining seated when required to do so
3. Is easily distracted by extraneous stimuli
4. Has difficulty awaiting turn in games or group situations
5. Often blurts out answers to questions before they have been completed
6. Has difficulty following through on instructions from others (not caused by oppositional behavior or failure of comprehension) (e.g., fails to finish chores)
7. Has difficulty sustaining attention in tasks or play activities
8. Often shifts from one uncompleted activity to another
9. Has difficulty playing quietly
10. Often talks excessively
11. Often interrupts or intrudes on others (e.g., butts into other children's games)
12. Often does not seem to listen to what is being said to him or her
13. Often loses things necessary for tasks or activities at school or at home (e.g., toys, pencils, books, assignments)
14. Often engages in physically dangerous activities without considering possible consequences (not for the purpose of thrill-seeking) (e.g., runs into street without looking)

Note: The above items are listed in descending order of discrimination power based on data from a national field trial of the DSM-IIIR criteria for Disruptive Behavior Disorders
B. Onset before the age of 7
C. Does not meet the criteria for a Pervasive Developmental Disorder

CRITERIA FOR SEVERITY OF ADHD

Mild: Few, if any, symptoms in excess of those required to make the diagnosis and only minimal or no impairment in school and social functioning
Moderate: Symptoms or functional impairment intermediate between "mild" and "severe."
Severe: Many symptoms in excess of those required to make the diagnosis and significant and pervasive impairment in functioning at home and school and with peers

of the syndrome is variable, some children being only mildly affected, whereas in others, the whole of the child's social life is disrupted by the severity of the disorder. There is excessive motor activity, the child's restlessness being manifested by difficulties in remaining seated for prolonged periods of time, excessive fidgetting, and a tendency to run around often quite inappropriately. These children are also impulsive, often being unable to postpone their speaking or motor activity until an appropriate moment, with associated lack of ability to remain attentive to subjects for the ordinary length of time. They have difficulty organizing their thinking with poor attention span and careless attention to detail.

There has been a considerable debate as to whether ADHD is a true medical syndrome, with a specific etiology, and a stable prognosis. It is reasonable to state that, in spite of DSM III and DSM IIIR, this at the present time is not settled, although the presentation of children with some of these behaviors is familiar to everyone. Follow-up studies suggest that the syndrome does continue in a proportion of patients into adolescence, such children showing poorer academic performance, difficult relationships with their peers, and an increase in antisocial behavior. Further, retrospective analyses of adults manifesting impulsivity, restlessness, or emotional lability reveal a subgroup that would have qualified for a diagnosis of ADHD as children.

There has been considerable literature on the treatment of hyperactivity syndromes with medications, most studies using central nervous system stimulants such as methylphenidate and amphetamine. There does not appear to be strict syndrome specificity, in the sense that children with other diagnoses have been shown responsive to these drugs, and only 70–80% of hyperactive children respond favorably. However, stimulants do improve concentration and performance in the classroom setting, and a tendency to aggressive behaviors and impulsivity is diminished. Follow-up studies do not confirm long-term benefits with regard to emotional or antisocial behavior, and school performance.

Other medications have been used in this syndrome, including tricyclic antidepressants, neuroleptics such as thioridazine and haloperidol, and anticonvulsants. Further, there is growing evidence that some anticonvulsants, in particular phenobarbitone, may precipitate or exacerbate hyperactive behavior, leading to an effect opposite to that of the stimulants.

The anticonvulsant most used in treatments has been carbamazepine, some authors reporting that small doses of only 50 mg once or twice a day lead to a reduction of symptoms. However, doses of up to 1,000 mg/day may be needed, authors gradually increasing the dose until a beneficial effect is noticed. The symptoms most responsive to carbamazepine appear to be aggressive behavior, hyperactivity, distractibility, low tolerance of frustration, and impulsiveness. As a consequence of the improved behavior, there is accelerated learning and better control in the classroom.

In a review paper on the use of carbamazepine in pediatric psychiatry, Evans and colleagues (1987) presented a case of their own with ADHD and learning disability with aggressive outbursts and temporal "epileptiform" spike activity on the EEG. A dramatic improvement of behavior was noted with 600–800 mg of carbamazepine daily. They concluded "carbamazepine may be indicated in virtually any kind of serious childhood disturbance that does not respond to ordinary firstline treatments."

Groh and colleagues (1975) carried out a double-blind crossover trial of 20 nonepileptic children with various patterns of behavior disorder, comparing carbamazepine with placebo. Carbamazepine was significantly better, children showing improvement of mood and drive, and a reduction of anxiety or neurotic symptoms. Aggressiveness and hyperkinesis were the symptoms that responded the best. They also reviewed long-term treatment in nonepileptic children with behavior disorders receiving carbamazepine and noted 43% to show continuing improvements, most notably in emotional lability, moodiness, and hyperkinesis.

In view of the association of the syndrome to minimal brain dysfunction, EEG abnormalities are not infrequently found in association. It is not clear from the literature whether children with these abnormalities are more likely to respond to anticonvulsants, although it is the impression of some authors that this indeed is the case.

Children with epilepsy not uncommonly display behavioral patterns that include ADHD. The most comprehensive epidemiological studies of behavior disturbances in children come from Rutter and colleagues (1970). Using the Isle of Wight population in the United Kingdom, 29% of 63 children with epilepsy, uncomplicated by other neurological disorders, had some psychiatric condition, compared to 7% in the general population sample. The rates were even higher for children with complicated epilepsy. Although the majority of the epileptic children showed a mixture of emotional and conduct disorders, similar in spectrum to those found in children without obvious brain damage, a few children showed rarer syndromes of hyperkinesis, often associated with a degree of mental retardation. There is evidence from the literature on epileptic children that in some cases, this syndrome is driven by some anticonvulsants, in particular phenobarbitone. For example, Wolf and Forsythe (1955) reported that 42% of 109 children treated daily with phenobarbitone for febrile convulsions developed a behavior disorder, usually hyperactivity. This often did not appear until several months after the prescription, was not correlated with serum barbiturate levels, and disappeared in the majority when the barbiturate therapy was discontinued.

Benzodiazepine anticonvulsants have a similar effect. Clonazepam is used widely in childhood seizure disorders as oral adjunctive therapy, particularly for absence attacks, infantile spasms, "minor motor seizures," and the Lennox-Gastaut syndrome. Behavior disorders are the most com-

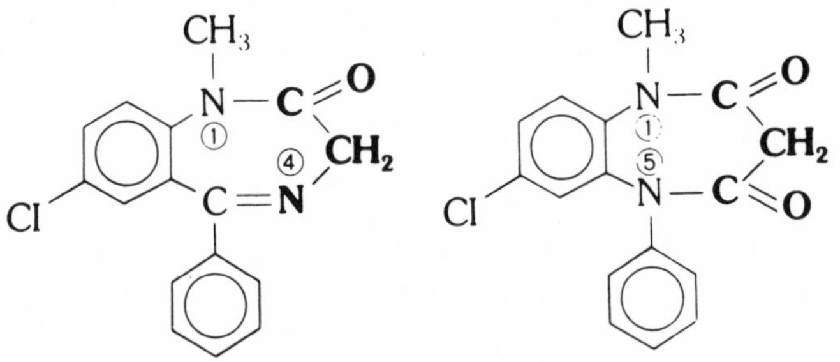

DIAZEPAM   CLOBAZAM

FIG. 6-1. Structure of the 1,4- compared with the 1,5-benzodiazepines.

monly reported side effects, aggressive behavior, irritability, disobedience, disinhibited behavior, and hyperactivity being commonly noted. The most recently introduced anticonvulsant drug, clobazam, which differs from the other benzodiazepines in being a 1,5-benzodiazepine, with its nitrogen radicals in positions 1 and 5, instead of 1 and 4, is less likely to provoke this effect (Fig. 6-1).

It is as yet unclear whether the anticonvulsants that are associated with ADHD merely exacerbate minor and tolerated behavior problems, or if they precipitate these states *de novo*. Clinically, the important point is to recognize the association and to avoid these drugs in such settings.

Conduct Disorder

The diagnostic criteria for conduct disorder are given in Table 6-2. The essential feature as given in DSM IIIR is "a persistent pattern of conduct in which the basic rights of others and major age-appropriate societal laws or norms are violated." As with ADHD, its nosological status is questioned, and there are clear overlaps with it. Aggressive outbursts are common to both conditions, as are poor self-esteem and academic underachievement. Some authors such as Quay and Quay (1965) would hold that the hyperkinetic syndrome exists separately from conduct disorder, noting clear differences on factor analytic studies, others such as Connors (1969) have failed to substantiate such claims.

Follow-up studies of children with ADHD reveal, in addition to the continuing attention-deficit disorder, a significant number of children who by adolescence develop conduct disorder or antisocial personality disorder. Further, the studies of Robins (1978) confirm that adult antisocial behavior is strongly associated with childhood antisocial behavior, although most antisocial children do not necessarily become antisocial adults.

Table 6-2. Diagnostic Criteria for Conduct Disorder

A. A disturbance of conduct lasting at least 6 months, during which at least three of the following have been present:
   1. Has stolen without confrontation of a victim on more than one occasion (including forgery)
   2. Has run away from home overnight at least twice while living in parental or parental surrogate home (or once without returning)
   3. Often lies (other than to avoid physical or sexual abuse)
   4. Has deliberately engaged in fire-setting
   5. Is often truant from school (for older person, absent from work)
   6. Has broken into someone else's house, building, or car
   7. Has deliberately destroyed others' property (other than by fire-setting)
   8. Has been physically cruel to animals
   9. Has forced someone into sexual activity with him or her
   10. Has used a weapon in more than one fight
   11. Often initiates physical fights
   12. Has stolen with confrontation of a victim (e.g., mugging, purse-snatching, extortion, armed robbery)
   13. Has been physically cruel to people

Note: The above items are listed in descending order of discriminating power based on data from a national field trial of the DMS-IIIR criteria for Disruptive Behavior Disorders

B. If 18 or older, does not meet criteria for Antisocial Personality Disorder

CRITERIA FOR SEVERITY OF CONDUCT DISORDER

Mild: Few if any conduct problems in excess of those required to make the diagnosis, and conduct problems cause only minor harm to others
Moderate: Number of conduct problems and effect on others intermediate between "mild" and "severe"
Severe: Many conduct problems in excess of those required to make the diagnosis, or conduct problems causing considerable harm to others (e.g., serious physical injury to victims, extensive vandalism or theft, prolonged absence from home)

In contrast to ADHD, there is little written on the medical treatment of conduct disorder, although anticonvulsants have a place. This literature includes studies of patients with epilepsy.

Although there is more general agreement that phenobarbitone influences behavior adversely, there have been few studies about this. Trimble and Corbett (1980) examined the association between behavior disorders and anticonvulsants in a population of children with intractable epilepsy using the parents' and teachers' behavior rating scales devised by Rutter to assess behavior problems. It was reported that 50% of the children on phenobarbitone had some form of conduct disturbance. No clear associations between phenytoin and conduct disorder emerged.

Ferrari and colleagues (1983) reported on 45 children with either epilepsy, diabetes, or no known health problems, some of whom were receiving barbiturate anticonvulsants. Children taking barbiturates had lower self-concept scores, and had more behavior problems at school. They more often displayed atypical behaviors including excessive worry, self-destructive behavior, and complaints of persecution.

There have been some studies about children being given anticonvulsants prophylactically for febrile convulsions. Heckmatt et al. (1976) noted that 16 of 88 patients using phenobarbitone developed behavior problems that subsequently improved in 12 when treatment stopped. Aldridge-Smith and Wallace (1982) gave 121 consecutive patients admitted for first convulsions either phenobarbitone or sodium valproate or no therapy. Parents were asked to rate their children's preconvulsive behavior with reassessment at 12 and 24 months later. There was no significant difference with regard to seizure frequency between the two drugs, but twice as many children on phenobarbitone deteriorated in at least one aspect of behavior in comparison with the sodium valproate group, whereas the parents of five reported improved behavior.

Carbamazepine has generally been reported to produce favorable reports on behavior, although adverse idiosyncratic behavior problems, including psychosis have been reported. Many of the systematic studies have been carried out on children with behavior disturbances, with or without EEG abnormalities, but often with no evidence of a seizure disorder. For example, de Weiss and colleagues (1974) investigated 33 children with disorders of conduct and EEG abnormalities. A double-blind comparison between carbamazepine (mean daily dose, 300 mg/day) and placebo was carried out. Behavior was evaluated by psychiatric and psychological interviews with each child and his parents. A statistically significant improvement in symptoms was found for the drug group in 15 of 17, compared to 8 of 16 in the placebo group. Likewise, Groh and colleagues (1975) carried out a double-blind crossover trial against placebo on 20 children of normal intelligence with a variety of behavior problems. The 6-week treatment periods were separated by a therapy-free interval of at least 4 weeks. Behavior was evaluated using a 39-item questionnaire completed by parents and teachers. There was a highly significant difference with respect to change noted on placebo and drug, the greater improvements being noted with the drug. A definite improvement was seen in 10 children, 6 showed a moderate improvement, and there was no change in 3. A deterioration was noted in one subject in the active compound group.

In the study of Trimble and Corbett (1980), serum levels of carbamazepine were correlated against scores on a conduct disorder rating scale in deviant children. A significant negative correlation emerged as shown in Fig. 6-2. In other words, the higher the level of carbamazepine, the lower the behavior-deviant score. This was significantly different from the noted effect of phenobarbitone.

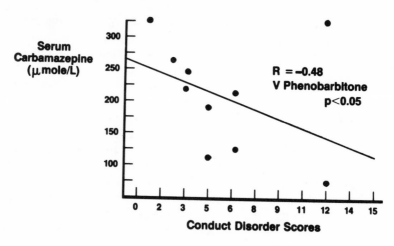

FIG. 6-2. Relationship between serum carbamazepine level and scores on a conduct disorder rating scale for children receiving anticonvulsant drugs is shown.

ANXIETY DISORDERS

DSM IIIR outlines a variety of anxiety disorders of childhood or adolescence including separation anxiety disorder, avoidance disorder, and overanxious disorder. There is not unnaturally some overlap with adult disorders, particularly in adolescence. The main anticonvulsants likely to be used in this setting are benzodiazepines, and there are several reports of the use of clonazepam in anxiety conditions, particularly with panic attacks. Symptoms are reported to be rapidly controlled, in daily doses ranging from 0.5 to 3 mg.

ANTICONVULSANT POLYTHERAPY, BEHAVIOR, AND COGNITIVE FUNCTION IN CHILDREN

There is at least a hint in the literature on epilepsy that polytherapy may bring adverse consequences for behavior and cognitive function in children, as it does in adults. Trimble and colleagues have completed a series of studies in which alteration of anticonvulsant prescriptions in children has been evaluated, the cognitive status of the children being rated using a series of microcomputer-delivered tests, and questionnaires being completed to assess behavior.

An automated test battery essentially examined perceptuomotor performance, attention and sensory processing, central cognitive processing, and memory. The behavior questionnaire used was the Connors Parent Symptom Questionnaire (CPSQ) and the Children's Depression Inventory (CDI).

This latter is a modification of the adult Beck Depression Inventory that allows children to assess their own mood.

Forty-four children with epilepsy, aged 7–17 years, and 21 nonepileptic children, aged 7–12 years, were assessed on three occasions over a period of 6 months, separated by 3-monthly intervals. The control group was compared with three subgroups of children as follows: the first remained on the same anticonvulsant regime throughout (N = 18); the second underwent a decrease in dose or number of drugs (N = 16); whereas the third had an increase in dose or number of drugs (N = 10). The three epilepsy groups were comparable with respect to age and full-scale IQ, which was within the average range. The normal control group had a significantly lower age and higher full-scale IQ, but these differences were covaried for in the statistical analysis. There was no significant change in seizure frequency for the three epilepsy groups over time.

In these investigations, clear differences were noted between the increase and decrease groups on a number of cognitive tasks and on the behavior questionnaire. Thus, increasing the antiepileptic drug load had a detrimental effect on the time taken to complete a task of simple perceptual identification of stimuli, and the time taken to access previously stored information. The decrease group, in contrast, showed improved performance on a face recognition task not exhibited by the other groups (Fig. 6-3). On the behavior questionnaire, the greatest improvement in score over time on the CPSQ was seen in the decrease group, both with regard to the total score and some subfactors such as conduct problems, anxiety, and learning problems. In particular, the children decreasing their anticonvulsant drug load showed a significant decrease in scores on the CDI, no changes in behavior on this or the CPSQ being noted in the group whose drug load was increased.

Differences Between Individual Anticonvulsant Drugs in Children

In this investigation, it was also possible to compare and contrast the performance over a 6-month interval of three groups of children taking different drug regimes. There was a group on polytherapy (N = 14), and a group on constant carbamazepine or sodium valproate monotherapy (N = 21). No difference in age of onset was found between these two groups, and after covarying for seizure frequency, several significant differences in favor of those on monotherapy were noted as shown in Table 6-3. Further, when children receiving carbamazepine monotherapy (N = 12) were compared with a group on sodium valproate monotherapy (N = 9), taking seizure frequency into account, some significant differences were noted, with respect to response latency, which favored carbamazepine. These tasks, shown in Table 6-4, included changes on reaction time tasks, a coding task, a digit-matching task, and a semantic memory task, mea-

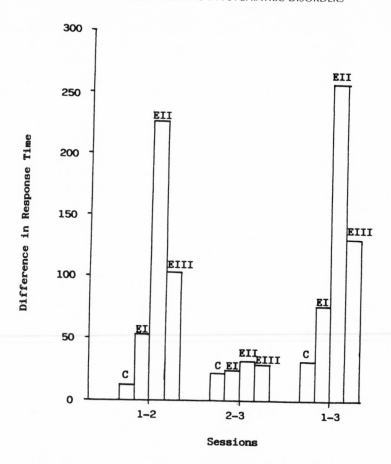

FIG. 6-3. Difference in response time on a minimum face-recognition memory task following change of medications in four groups of children. C, nonepileptic controls; EI, epileptic children, no drug change; EII, epileptic children who are decreasing their anticonvulsant drugs; EIII, children increasing their anticonvulsant drugs. The sessions are: (1) testing before change; (2) at 3 months; (3) at 6 months. The EII group shows significant improvements over time.

Table 6-3. Significant Differences (in Response Latency) between Children Receiving Polytherapy and Those on Monotherapy with either Carbamazepine or Sodium Valproate

Reaction time (three tasks)
Coding
Digit matching
Immediate recognition memory for faces
Perceptual identification
Semantic memory (i.e., accessing previously stored information)

Table 6-4. Response Latency Differences between Children on Carbamazepine and Sodium Valproate Monotherapy in Cognitive Function Studies

Reaction time (two tasks)
Coding task
Digit matching
Semantic memory (i.e., accessing previously stored information)

suring time taken to access previously stored information. When differences between the groups with regard to behavior measures were analyzed, no significant differences were noted. Interestingly, on the CDI, the only group to show changes over time was the carbamazepine group, which showed a significant decrease in score over the 6-month interval of the investigation.

The overall impression from these studies of children with epilepsy and from clinical experience is that carbamazepine is more often associated with minimal changes of behavior, and in this regard can be contrasted with the adverse effects of phenobarbitone. Polytherapy is more likely to be associated with problems than monotherapy.

In spite of this, there are anecdotal reports of occasional deterioration of behavior in patients receiving carbamazepine. The relationship of this to the carbamazepine-epoxide metabolite has recently been considered. Although not specifically including the variety of behavior disorders discussed here, Schoeman and colleagues (1984) noted highly significant differences between plasma carbamazepine-epoxide values in patients with and without a variety of drug side effects, and a lowering of the level of the epoxide with alteration of therapy, for example by achieving monotherapy, led to disappearance of the problems in some children.

Table 6-5. Summary of the Effects of Anticonvulsant Drugs on Childhood Behavior

Drug	Effect
Carbamazepine	Psychotropic
Clobazam	Psychotropic
Clonazepam	Associated with conduct disorder and hyperactivity
Ethosuximide	?
Phenobarbitone	Associated with conduct disorder and hyperactivity
Phenytoin	Minimal
Primidone	? (breaks down to phenobarbitone)
Valproic acid	Minimal

In conclusion, the use of anticonvulsant drugs for behavior disturbances in children has been quite commonplace in clinical practice, and their effects on behavior have been studied, especially in epileptic children. Generally, favorable reports are noted for carbamazepine, in particular in relationship to aggressive disorders, conduct disorders, and in hyperactive impulsive syndromes. Although carbamazepine is not the drug of choice in ADHD, there is some suggestion that children with this condition will respond. Few other anticonvulsants have been used in the nonepileptic setting, although benzodiazepines, and particularly clonazepam, have been associated with improvement of anxiety-related conditions. The epilepsy literature also contrasts the adverse effects of phenobarbitone with the psychotropic influences of carbamazepine, both on mood and behavior, in particular phenobarbitone, exacerbating hyperactive and conduct disorders. In patients with these behavior problems, drugs such as the barbiturates should be avoided. A summary of the influence of anticonvulsant drugs on behavior in children is given in Table 6-5.

REFERENCES AND SUGGESTED READING

Castano GR. Uzo de carbamazepina en ninos con trasternos de la conducta. *Prensa Med Mex* 1972;37:215–220.

Connors CK. A teacher rating scale for use in drug studies in children. *Am J Psychiatry* 1969;126:152–156.

de Weiss MM, de Monk CG, Chardon MC, Waitz A. Entoque diagnostico y therapeutico del nino turbulento. *Sem Med* 1974;144:9–15.

Evans RW, Clay TH, Gualtiere CT. Carbamazepine in paediatric psychiatry. *J Am Acad Child Psychiatry* 1987;26:2–8.

Ferrari M, Barabas G, Matthews WS. Psychologic and behavioral disturbance among epileptic children treated with barbiturate anticonvulsants. *Am J Psychiatry* 1983;140:112–113.

Gastaut H, Low MD. Antiepileptic properties of clobazam, a 1,5-benzodiazepine, in man. *Epilepsia* 1980;20:437–446.

Gittelman R, Mannuzza S, Shenker R, Bonagura N. Hyperactive boys almost grown up. *Arch Gen Psychiatry* 1985;42:935–947.

Groh C. The psychotropic effect of tegretol in nonepileptic children. In: Birkmayer W, ed. *Epileptic Seizures—Behavior—Pain*. Berne: Hans Huber, 1975:259–263.

Heckmatt JK, Houston AB, Clow DJ, Stevenson JBP, Dodd KL, Lealman GT, Logan RW. Failure of phenobarbitone to prevent febrile convulsions. *Br Med J* 1976;1:559–561.

Herranz JL, Arteaga R, Armijo JA. Side effects of sodium valproate in monotherapy controlled by plasma levels: a study of 88 paediatric patients. *Epilepsia* 1982;23:203–214.

Kahn E, Cohen LH. Organic drivenness—a brain stem syndrome and an experience with case reports. *N Engl J Med* 1934;210:748–756.

Laufer MW, Denhoff E, Solomons G. Hyperkinetic impulse disorder in children with behaviour problems. *Psychosom Med* 1956;19:38–49.

Quay HC, Quay LC. Behaviour problems in early adolescence. *Child Dev* 1965;36:215–220.

Robins LN. Sturdy childhood predictors of adult antisocial behaviour: replications from longitudinal studies. *Psychol Med* 1978;8:611–622.

Rutter M, Graham P, Yule W. A neuropsychiatric study in childhood. *Clinics in Developmental Medicine Nos 35-36*. London: Heinemann Medical Books, 1970.

Schoeman JF, Elyas AA, Brett EM, Lascelles PT. Altered ration of carbamazepine 10,11-epoxide/carbamazepine in plasma of children. *Dev Med Child Neurol* 1984;26:749–755.

Trimble MR, Corbett J. Behavioural and cognitive disturbances in epileptic children. *Ir Med J* (suppl) 1980;73:21–28.

Weiss G, Kruger E, Danielson U, Elman M. The effect of long term treatment of hyperactive children with methylphenidate. *Can Med Assoc J* 1975;112:159–165.

Wender PH, Reimherr FW, Wood DR. Attention deficit disorder in adults. *Arch Gen Psychiatry* 1981;38:449–456.

Werry J, Aman M. Methylphenidate and haloperidol in children: effects on attention, memory and activity. *Arch Gen Psychiatry* 1975;32:790–795.

Wolf SM, Forsythe A. Behaviour disturbance, phenobarbital and febrile seizures. *Pediatrics* 1955;61:728–731.

7

Use of Anticonvulsants in the Treatment of Manic-Depressive Illness

Robert M. Post

ELECTROCONVULSIVE THERAPY AS THE FIRST WIDELY USED ANTICONVULSANT

Anticonvulsants have been used for almost a half century in the treatment of affective illness. The major motor seizures produced by electroconvulsive therapy (ECT) have profound anticonvulsant consequences clinically and in animal model systems. Repeated induction of electroconvulsive shock (ECS) seizures in man gradually increases the seizure threshold, in some instances to the point where patients become refractory to seizure induction and in other instances, in proportion to the degree of clinical efficacy of the treatment. ECS seizures in animals are effective both in preventing the development of amygdala-kindled seizures and in exerting long-lasting anticonvulsant effects once these seizures have been expressed. With a variety of recent technical advances, seizures for clinical treatment are induced under anesthesia in the presence of muscle relaxants and close physiological monitoring such that the process is performed in an atmosphere of surgical aesthetics and precision. This is very different from the popular image derived from early treatment applications without anesthesia and that portrayed in some movies such as *One Flew Over the Cuckoo's Nest.*

Recently, the efficacy of ECT in the treatment of acute depression has been reconfirmed in a series of double-blind trials against sham ECT. Moreover, studies of the comparative efficacy of ECT and more traditional psychopharmacological antidepressant modalities (such as the tricyclics) consistently demonstrate more favorable results for ECT. This is all the more the case in the treatment of acute delusional psychotic depression, which is notoriously refractory to treatment with antidepressant drugs but responds in a high proportion of cases to ECT. Thus, for the delusionally depressed patient, one with uncontrolled suicidal urges, and one with varieties of medical problems that might make pharmacotherapy inadvisable, ECT may remain a treatment of high priority if not the first choice. The details of the application of ECT will not be dealt with in this volume as they are adequately described elsewhere.

Older clinical observations and a series of more recent studies have indicated that bilateral ECT may also be effective in the treatment of acute mania. The mechanism responsible for the anticonvulsant effects of ECT remains to be elucidated, as do those mediating its psychotropic efficacy. Recent studies raise the possibility that ECT releases many peptides, including endogenous opiate peptides, into the cerebrospinal fluid (CSF) of animals; when CSF is transferred to other animals, a naloxone-reversible principle appears to mediate anticonvulsant effects. Because ECT affects a variety of other neurotransmitter and neuropeptide modulator systems, it is unclear whether its psychotropic properties are directly related to those mediating its anticonvulsant effects. ECT is an entirely experimental approach to the long-term treatment of recurrent manic-depressive illness, as systematic studies of efficacy in prophylaxis have not been reported.

CARBAMAZEPINE

The anticonvulsant carbamazepine is, after ECT, the next most well-studied anticonvulsant in the treatment of manic-depressive illness. Emerging evidence suggests that it shares a profile of clinical efficacy very similar to that of lithium carbonate where there is considerable evidence for acute efficacy in the treatment of mania, less data regarding its efficacy in acute depression, and an emerging clinical consensus that carbamazepine plays a role in the long-term prophylaxis of both manic and depressive episodes.

Although there is some similarity of clinical profile between lithium and carbamazepine, there are obvious major differences. In contrast to lithium, carbamazepine is a highly effective anticonvulsant, and it is also used clinically in the treatment of paroxysmal pain syndromes such as trigeminal neuralgia. Preliminary data suggest that different subgroups of patients with manic-depressive illness may show differential responsivity to lithium versus carbamazepine. The two drugs clearly have very different side-effect profiles and may have both similarities and differences in their mechanisms of action.

Carbamazepine in Acute Mania

As of August 1988, more than 10 double-blind studies have documented the acute antimanic efficacy of carbamazepine or its congeners in

the treatment of acute mania compared to either placebo, lithium, or neuroleptics. The incidence and time-course of antimanic effects of carbamazepine appear comparable with those achieved with neuroleptics, although several studies have suggested a slightly faster onset of efficacy of
neuroleptics in the first 3 days of treatment, a difference that was gone
by 7 days. Patients requiring seclusion for acute, fulminant, psychotic manic
episodes may rapidly improve following double-blind initiation of treatment with carbamazepine alone (Fig. 7-1).

Possible clinical predictors of positive response to carbamazepine have
been examined in 12 patients who improved, compared with the 7 who
showed little evidence of response. Those who improved were significantly more manic at onset, tended to be more dysphoric (higher depression ratings during their manias), were significantly more rapid cycling in
the year before admission to the National Institute of Mental Health
(NIMH), and tended to be overrepresented in the group with a negative
family history of affective illness in first-degree relatives (Table 7-1). Thus
it appears that many of the same variables that tend to be associated with
relatively poor response to lithium (i.e., manic severity, dysphoria, rapid
cycling, and negative family history of affective illness) may be variables
that are associated with a relatively good acute and/or longer-term prophylactic response to carbamazepine. It was also observed that sleep im-

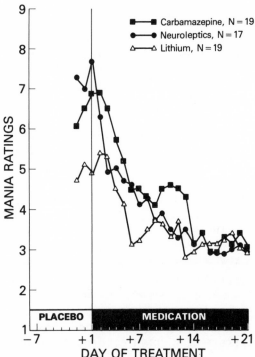

FIG 7-1. Time-course of antimanic effects of carbamazepine
compared to lithium and neuroleptics.

Table 7-1.   Predictors of Antimanic Response to Carbamazepine

Severity of Mania	Nonresponders (7)	Responders (12)	p
Base-line mania ratings	3.4 ± 0.8	8.0 ± 0.4	0.0001
Severity of manic dysphoria			
Base-line depression ratings (during manic episode)	4.5 ± 0.8	6.2 ± 0.5	0.10
Rapid cycling			
Episodes/years ill	1.2 ± 0.3	4.4 ± 1.7	0.10
Episodes in year prior to NIMH admission	2.7 ± 0.9	7.0 ± 1.6	0.03
Nonpredictors			
Age of onset, first treatment	21.0 ± 1.9	21.0 ± 1.7	NS
Duration of illness (years)	15.0 ± 4.6	18.0 ± 3.3	NS

proved within the first week of treatment (Fig. 7-2), and this occurred more robustly in responders compared to nonresponders.

In light of the data suggesting equal incidence of antimanic effects of carbamazepine compared with neuroleptics, and in view of the fact that neuroleptics produce uncomfortable acute parkinsonian side effects in a proportion of patients and that bipolar patients appear to be at particular risk for the development of tardive dyskinesia, it is suggested that the use of carbamazepine in place of a neuroleptic in the adjunctive treatment of the acute manic patient who is being initiated on lithium treatment be considered. Similarly, in the patient with acute mania breaking through lithium treatment, a clinical trial with carbamazepine and, sequentially, other anticonvulsants if necessary, may be advisable.

Moreover, if carbamazepine is tried instead of a neuroleptic, it may give valuable clinical information regarding acute efficacy that might also provide a helpful guideline for later consideration of what drugs may be useful in long-term prophylaxis of recurrent episodes. In addition, if a neuroleptic is not used or is used only sparingly in the acute treatment of a manic episode, then it is less likely to be continued unnecessarily during prophylaxis, thus lessening the risk of protracted neuroleptic treatment and the appearance of tardive dyskinesia. Even if neuroleptics are used exclusively and successfully in the adjunctive treatment of the acute manic episode, questions will remain unresolved regarding the agents that should be employed in subsequent prophylaxis. This is particularly the case for the lithium refractory patient whose manic episodes emerge in spite of concurrent lithium treatment. Thus, use of information regarding a pos-

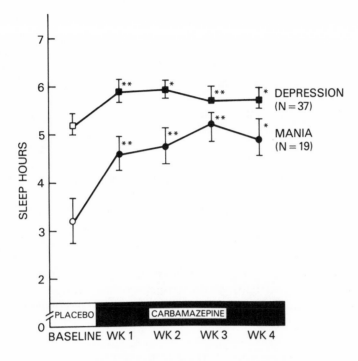

FIG. 7-2. Improvement in sleep during carbamazepine treatment.

itive or negative *acute* response to anticonvulsant adjuncts (carbamaze-pine, valproate, clonazepam) may help direct long-term prophylactic treatment.

It is suggested that carbamazepine treatment in acute mania be started at doses of 400–600 mg/day. These are higher than doses used when initiating treatment of an euthymic or depressed patient, when one should proceed much more slowly (see below). In mania, doses can be rapidly increased (by 200 mg/day) until a clinical response is observed or a maxi-mum of 1,600–1,800 mg/day is achieved. Dose increases should be ti-trated against the appearance of clinical side effects such as sedation, ataxia, dysarthria, or diplopia. There is a wide individual range at which these side effects occur, and physicians should adjust dosages individually rather than attempting to use an average dose or a hypothetical therapeutic win-dow.

Little evidence has been found of a relationship between blood levels for carbamazepine in the range of 4–12 μg/ml and the degree of anti-manic or antidepressant efficacy of the drug. Thus, titration to side ef-fects appears the most reasonable clinical approach. If a patient shows no evidence of acute antimanic response after several weeks at moderate doses and blood levels, it is unlikely that pushing the dose to toxicity will result in the onset of therapeutic effects (i.e., there does not appear to be a distinct threshold effect). In these instances, switching to another agent may be indicated. If, however, there is some evidence of clinical response initially, increasing the dose may be helpful, as a dose-related improvement in mania and psychosis in individual patients has been observed. Moreover, as carbamazepine induces its own hepatic metabolism, doses not tolerated in the first several weeks may be well accepted after 2 or 3 weeks of chronic administration.

A similar, although perhaps slightly less aggressive, dose management regimen can be considered in the adjunctive treatment of carbamazepine with lithium carbonate. Although there have been isolated reports of neurotoxicity from the two drugs used in combination, many of these effects appear attributable to the initiation of treatment with a high dose of carbamazepine. With slow dose titration, neurotoxic side effects of the lithium-carbamazepine combination are infrequent. Yet, they have been documented in selected patients and those most at risk may include patients with organic processes such as EEG abnormalities and histories of medical and neurological problems. Various aspects of the clinical laboratory profile of the lithium-carbamazepine interaction will be discussed in following sections.

Carbamazepine Treatment in Acute Depression

Post and colleagues have studied the effects of carbamazepine in 47 acutely depressed patients using a B-A-B double-blind substitution of carbamazepine for placebo. Fifteen of the 47 patients have shown substantial degrees of improvement, with most of these patients showing a change sufficient to enable them to be discharged from the hospital (Fig. 7-3). Although this approximately 32% response rate does not appear very high, it should be noted that it is occurring in patients who were otherwise treatment refractory and were referred to NIMH as a tertiary referral center. Moreover, response occurred after patients had had extensive periods of placebo evaluation while they were hospitalized, such that placebo responders had already been eliminated from the cohort. Nonetheless, other clinical trials are clearly needed in order to establish the relative efficacy of carbamazepine compared with other agents in randomized designs.

Most of the patients included in that series were bipolar and the degree of responsivity to carbamazepine in unipolar depressed patients remains to be delineated. To date, 2 of 15 unipolar depressed patients have responded. In light of this meager evidence and in the face of a whole series of very effective and proven treatment modalities for the unipolar depressed patient, carbamazepine would not be placed as high in the series of treatment options for the unipolar depressed patients as it would for

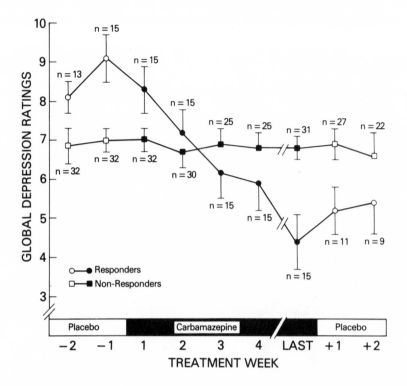

FIG. 7-3. Antidepressant course in patients with marked response to carbamazepine.

the bipolar depressed patient. In bipolar illness, carbamazepine is a first-line treatment option after lithium and a potential supplement in patients with bipolar illness breaking through lithium treatment. A differential sequence of treatments in the unipolar compared to the bipolar depressed patient is schematized in Table 7-2. Note this sequence is highly provisional and the order should be revised and tailored to each individual patient's presenting symptoms, course of illness, and past medical history.

In a preliminary analysis, several interesting clinical predictors of an antidepressant response emerged (Post et al., 1986b). Again, those with more severe depression at the outset were among those who responded best to carbamazepine (see Fig. 7-3). Responders showed the usual lag in onset of antidepressant efficacy with little evidence of improvement in the first and second weeks of treatment but with considerable improvement by the fourth, fifth, and sixth weeks (see Fig. 7-3). It is important that this lag in onset of antidepressant effects of carbamazepine be considered, particularly in relationship to the apparently more rapid onset of acute antimanic effects. In contrast to the treatment of acute mania, where if there is no evidence of antimanic effects by the end of the second or third

Table 7-2. Differential Sequence of Treatments in Depression Subtypes[a]

Unipolar depression	vs.	Bipolar depression
1. Tricyclic or heterocyclic No. 1		1. Lithium
2. Tricyclic or heterocyclic No. 2		1A. Plus carbamazepine
2A. Plus T_3 potentiation		2. Carbamazepine
2B. or lithium potentiation		2A. Plus lithium
2C. or sleep deprivation poten-		2B. Triple combination
tiation		—Thyroid or,
2–4. MAOI (atypicality)		—MAOI or,
2–5. Lithium (recurrent, bipolar family		—Tricyclic
history)		3. Valproic acid
3–4. Alprazolam (mild with panic)		4. Calcium channel blockers
6. Carbamazepine (recurrent)		5. Clonazepam
7. Bromocriptine		6. Buprorion
8. Tricyclic-MAOI Combination??		7. Spironolactone
9. Psychomotor stimulants (a.m.		8. Tryptophan or 5-HTP
retardation)		
10. Tryptophan or 5-HTP (insomnia;		1–3. Tricyclic or MAOI
low 5-HIAA)		
1–10. ECT (depending on severity and		1–8. — (ECT)
medical and suicidal risk)		
(1). Plus neuroleptics (for delusional		1. Plus neuroleptic (delusional)
depression)		
Chlorimipramine (for obses-		
sional disorder)		
Light (seasonal)		
1–10. Revision in type of psychother-		1–10. Revision in type of psychother-
apy		apy

[a] ECT, electroconvulsive therapy; 5-HTP, 5-hydroxytryptophan; 5-HIAA, 5-hydrox-
yindoleacetic acid; MAOI, monoamine oxidase inhibitor; T_3, triiodothyronine.

week of treatment the use of carbamazepine might be abandoned for other
agents, it would behoove the clinician to continue treatment of the depressed patient for some longer period of time. Patients who had a prior
history of more discrete episodes and less chronic depression were also
among those who responded. Improvement in sleep (based on nurses'
half-hourly sleep checks) occurred in the first week of treatment (see Fig.
7-2) and was dissociated from the degree of subsequent antidepressant
responses (i.e., improvement in sleep was not correlated with improvement in mood). Paradoxically, those patients who showed the greatest degree of decreases in thyroxine (T_4) and free T_4 showed the greatest degree of clinical improvement $(r = -.50, N=38$, and $r = -.56, N=36, p<.001)$.
The effects of carbamazepine on thyroid indices will be further discussed
below.

Several pertinent factors that did not correlate with the degree of anti-depressant responses are noteworthy. It was not found that even minor EEG changes (within the range of normal) were associated with clinical response. Patients with manic-depressive illness have a high incidence of psychosensory symptoms similar to those reported by patients with complex partial seizures. These include not only common phenomena such as deja vu but a variety of alterations in sensory experiences, visual and olfactory illusions, and the like. To be considered a psychosensory symptom, occurrence must be paroxysmal, last a brief period of time (a matter of seconds to minutes), and not be attributable to any other outside factor such as ingestion of a drug or physical illness. Silberman et al. (1985) had hoped that these symptoms, which have been considered a marker of temporal lobe dysfunction (they are often reported by patients whose temporal lobe and limbic systems are electrically stimulated), might provide a predictor of which patients would respond to the limbic anticonvulsant, carbamazepine. Disappointingly, they found no such relationship between the occurrence of these psychosensory symptoms and the degree of response to carbamazepine (Fig. 7-4) and, on the contrary, found that those who showed the best responses to lithium carbonate had the highest number of psychosensory symptoms. Thus, although the clinician might use findings of minor EEG abnormalities or a history of psychosensory phenomena as a justification for considering the use of an anticonvulsant in patients with primary affective illness, it should be recognized that there

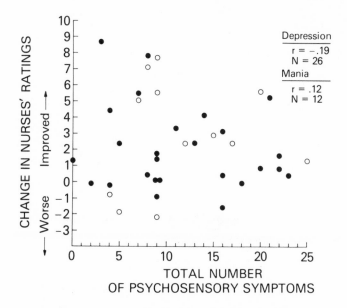

FIG. 7-4. Psychosensory symptoms do not predict antidepressant (●) or antimanic (○) responses to carbamazepine.

is little evidence of such a relationship with these factors. This is not to say that patients with clear-cut evidence of complex partial seizures do not show excellent psychotropic responses to treatment with carbamazepine, but that responses can occur independently of EEG or psychosensory changes (see Fig. 7-4).

Among the two-thirds of patients who were inadequately responsive to treatment with carbamazepine alone, Kramlinger and Post (1989) observed that 8 of 15 patients (53%) given supplemental treatment with lithium carbonate on a blind basis showed a rapid onset of antidepressant responses (Fig. 7-5). These data are very similar to those in which lithium potentiation has been used with more traditional tricyclic, heterocyclic,

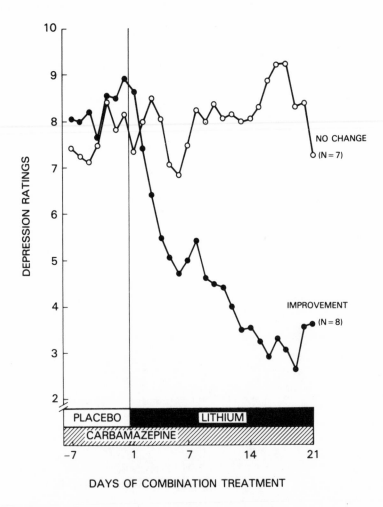

FIG. 7-5. Lithium potentiation in nonresponders to carbamazepine.

and monoamine oxidase inhibitor antidepressants. Similar to the original reports of DeMontigny and associates (1981) in Canada, Kramlinger and Post (1989) observed that the antidepressant effects of lithium potentiation tended to be rather rapid, often occurring in the first 2–4 days of treatment (Fig. 7-5). This effect was more rapid than that seen in patients responding to the antidepressant effects of lithium carbonate alone, and was even more rapid than those showing response to lithium potentiation of carbamazepine-inadequate response in acute mania. These data suggest that the mechanism of lithium potentiation of antidepressant effects is different from that observed with lithium treatment alone (it may involve the serotonin system) and also provide the interesting clinical message that if response is not observable within the first 1 to 3 weeks of lithium potentiation for an acute episode, it is not likely to occur.

Based on the wealth of clinical data suggesting that some 60% of patients reported in the literature may show a positive response to lithium potentiation of previously ineffective antidepressant modalities, it is suggested that this potentiation treatment be used earlier in the sequence of antidepressant modalities than one might usually consider. That is, as illustrated in Table 7-2, during the first or second trial of a heterocyclic agent, one might consider potentiation first with triiodothyronine (T_3) and then with lithium carbonate rather than rotating the patient to the next drug with the attendant risks of continued nonresponse and a likely wait of at least 3 to 6 weeks before this response is adequately delineated and blood levels are optimized. If the patient does show a response to thyroid or lithium potentiation, a considerable amount of time would thus be conserved. For the unipolar depressed patient, lack of response to a tricyclic might also suggest the utility of shifting to a monoamine oxidase inhibitor (MAOI) antidepressant, as recent evidence suggests that many unipolar patients who fail an initial trial with tricyclics will respond to the MAOIs. Switching to the selective serotonin reuptake blockers fluoxetine and cloimipramine might also be considered, as might the triazolobenzodiazepine alprazolam in cases with a high degree of anxiety. It would not generally be prudent to use carbamazepine until a variety of these more traditional and approved modalities had been used in the treatment of the unipolar depressed patient.

In contrast, carbamazepine is much higher on the list of treatments for the bipolar patient in part because of the increasing (but still controversial) concerns regarding tricyclic and MAOI precipitation of mania, induction of rapid cycling, or conversion to a pattern of continuous cycling between mania and depression without a well interval. Although estimates of the ability of these agents to switch patients into mania usually range from 8 to 15%, in bipolar patients this may rise to one-fourth or one-third of patients. It is also clear that in relatively rapid cycling patients, the addition of a tricyclic may speed up the frequency of cycling, which upon drug discontinuation may return to base-line. Thus, for the bipolar patient, and particularly one with severe episodes of prior mania or a history of rapid cycling, the addition of carbamazepine to lithium might be considered (or vice versa if the person is not already treated with lithium) in preference to a typical antidepressant. Again, if acute antidepressant response is achieved with carbamazepine, the efficacy of a mood stabilizer might help resolve decisions about subsequent drugs to be used in prophylaxis. If the bipolar patient does not respond acutely to the combination of lithium and carbamazepine, a tricyclic or MAOI can be added to the treatment regimen in the hope (not yet tested systematically) that the two antimanic and anticycling agents concurrently used would prevent tricyclic-induced rapid cycling. If used in this fashion, when the acute episode is over, the tricyclic or MAOI should be discontinued as soon as possible.

Clinical Laboratory Effects of Carbamazepine and Lithium

Because lithium carbonate and carbamazepine may be used in combination for acute and prophylactic treatment of manic and depressive illness, it is reasonable to consider the side effects of carbamazepine alone and in combination with lithium carbonate. The differential side-effect profiles of the two drugs is outlined in Table 7-3. The side effects that tend to be problematic during treatment with lithium are often not a problem on carbamazepine. These include polydipsia and polyuria (as part of the diabetes insipidus [DI] syndrome), tremor, gastrointestinal disturbances, complaints of cognitive slowing, and weight gain. In contrast to lithium, carbamazepine has been used to treat DI, although when the two drugs are used in combination, the effects of lithium will override those of carbamazepine, and carbamazepine will not be able to reduce or prevent lithium-induced DI. This is because carbamazepine appears to act at or close to the vasopressin receptor, whereas lithium carbonate appears to exert its effects below the vasopressin receptor at the level of inhibition of adenylate cyclase. Thus, carbamazepine may be an alternative agent which will not produce DI, but it will not reverse lithium-induced DI. To the extent that complaints of cognitive slowing and impairment in learning and memory on lithium are also attributable to its ability to block vasopressin function (in brain, rather than kidney), the previous analysis would suggest that carbamazepine might not share this same side effect, but it would be unable to reverse lithium's effects. As reviewed in Chapter 2, carbamazepine appears to have the most benign side effects on cognitive function among the anticonvulsants. Systematic tests exploring the cognitive effects of carbamazepine compared to lithium have just been initiated. Two preliminary studies suggest equal and insignificant effects of both drugs on a variety of cognitive tests, but perhaps more sensitive tests are required.

Table 7-3. Comparative Clinical and Side-Effect Profiles of Lithium and Carbamazepine

	Lithium	Carbamazepine	Lithium-carbamazepine combination
Clinical profile[a]			
Mania	+ +	+ +	+ + +
Dysphoric	+	+	+ +
Rapid cycling	+	+ +	+ +
Continuous cycling	+	+	+ +
Family history negative	+	+ +	+ + +
Depression	+	+	+ + +
Prophylaxis of mania and depression	+ +	+ +	+ + +
Epilepsy	0	+ +	?
Pain syndromes	0	+ +	?
Side effects[b]			
White blood count	↑	↓	(↑), Li*
DI[c]	↑	↓	↑, Li*
Thyroid hormones T_3, T_4[c]	↓	↓	↓ ↓
TSH[c]	↑	–	↑, Li*
Serum calcium	(↑)	↓	
Weight gain	(↑)	–	
Tremor	(↑)	–	
Memory disturbances	(↑)	?	
Diarrhea	(↑)	–	
Teratogenesis	(↑)	–	
Psoriasis	(↑)	–	
Pruritic rash (allergy)	–	↑	
Agranulocytosis	–	(↑)	
Hepatitis	–	(↑)	
Hyponatremia, water intoxication	–	(↑)	
Dizziness, ataxia, diplopia	–	↑	
Hypercortisolism, escape from dexamethasone suppression	–	↑	

[a]Clinical efficacy: 0, none; +, effective; + +, very effective; + + +, possible synergism.

[b]Side effects: ↑, increase; ↓, decrease; ( ), inconsistent or rare; –, absent; ↓ ↓, potentiation; Li*, effect of lithium predominates.

[c]DI, diabetes insipidus; T_3, triiodothyronine; T_4, thyroxine; TSH, thyroid-stimulating hormone.

Another area where the effects of lithium and carbamazepine are opposite is on hematological indices. Lithium is well known for its ability to increase the white count by stimulating colony-stimulating factors for the granulocytic and megakaryocytic series in the bone marrow. In contrast, it has recently been demonstrated by Gallicchio and Hulette (1989) that carbamazepine suppresses these two factors. This accounts for its ability to typically induce benign white cell suppression in the majority of patients in whom it is used. When the two drugs are used in combination, the effects of lithium override those of carbamazepine, but in a clinically useful manner.

As illustrated in Fig. 7-6, not only does lithium potentiation reverse the white count suppression of carbamazepine, but values return above those of base line. Even though carbamazepine does not decrease base-line platelet counts, the positive effect of lithium is still evident when the two drugs are used in combination. Thus, in instances when the absolute white count is in the range of 1,500 cells/cm, and lithium potentiation might otherwise be indicated for clinical reasons, it appears reasonable to consider augmenting treatment with lithium in order to increase white cells toward normal. This should be attempted only when the other hematological indices are within normal limits. This is apparent because lithium is able to reverse the benign white count suppression of carbamazepine, but it is highly doubtful that it would be able to reverse the more problematic idiosyncratic processes of agranulocytosis or aplastic anemia. In particular, if the red count or hematocrit is abnormal, one should immediately

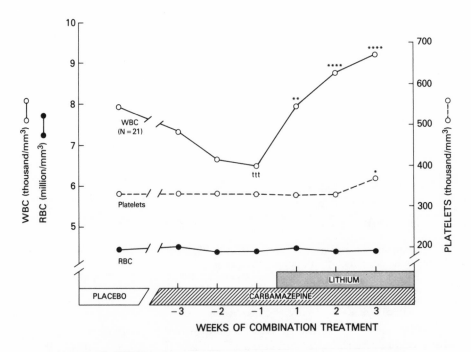

FIG. 7-6. Hematological indices during lithium potentiation of carbamazepine.

discontinue carbamazepine as lithium will not stimulate the colony-stimulating factors for the red cell series.

Thus, two distinctly different hematological effects of carbamazepine should be distinguished. One is the benign white count suppression where values may decrease into the range of 3,000–4,000 cells/cm. In the absence of changes in other indices, this would not appear problematic. This common effect appears to be reversible by lithium carbonate. In contrast, aplastic anemia and agranulocytosis appear to occur on the order of 8 cases per million or 1 in 125,000 (Pellock, 1987). As these very rare idiosyncratic reactions can emerge suddenly, it is doubtful that frequent hematological monitoring is indicated once it is established that carbamazepine is not acutely inducing serious hematological suppression. Certainly warning patients to call their physician and have a complete blood count is indicated if they should develop a fever, sore throat, rash, petechiae, or other evidence of a hematological or bleeding disorder.

Carbamazepine and lithium exert differential effects on thyroid indices. Both drugs decrease circulating levels of T_4, free T_4, and T_3. However, only lithium produces significant increases in thyroid-stimulating hormone (TSH) levels and clinically relevant hypothyroidism which requires thyroid replacement in a small but significant proportion of patients. When the two drugs are used in combination, the suppression in thyroid indices are additive, yet the increase in TSH observed is similar to that observed with lithium alone (Fig. 7-7). In light of the data mentioned above that the degree of decrease in free T_4 and T_4 is correlated with the degree of acute antidepressant efficacy of carbamazepine and the virtual lack of reports of carbamazepine-induced hypothyroidism, periodic measurement of thyroid function during lithium treatment, but not necessarily carbamazepine, is recommended. When the two drugs are used in combination, one should again attend to the potential lithium-induced effects on thyroid function and the associated need for thyroid replacement.

Because thyroid potentiation has been reported to be effective in a moderate percentage of acutely depressed patients refractory to traditional antidepressant agents, we would recommend a clinical trial of T_3 potentiation even in the face of normal thyroid indices. Use of 25–50 μg of T_3 rather than T_4 are recommended for this acute potentiation, as recent data from Joffe et al. (1989) suggest that it is more effective than T_4, raising the theoretical possibility that T_3 potentiation may in part be acting by suppressing circulating levels of T_4 like carbamazepine and lithium. Plasma T_4 is actively and selectively taken up in the brain and converted intercellularly to T_3. In contrast, when replacing thyroid for lithium-induced hypothyroidism, T_4 is usually recommended because of its longer half-life and smoother therapeutic action than T_3. Doses should be titrated upward very slowly, however, as steady-state levels may not be reached for some period of time (1–2 weeks) and should hyperthyroidism

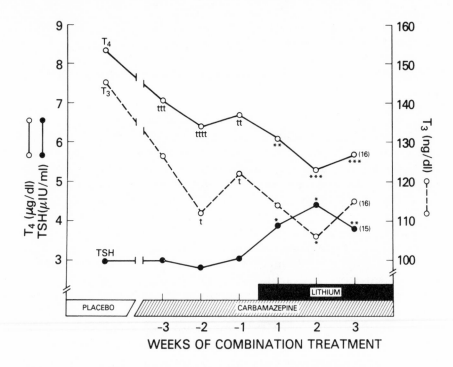

FIG. 7-7. Thyroid indices during lithium potentiation of carbamazepine.

supervene, it cannot be as rapidly reversed by withdrawing T_4 as it is by withdrawing T_3. Either T_3 or T_4 has been used in thyroid potentiation of the prophylactic effects of lithium, carbamazepine, or their combination, as discussed below.

Although carbamazepine's ability to decrease serum calcium is statistically significant, it does not appear to be of clinical relevance and does not require routine clinical monitoring. In contrast, carbamazepine may induce degrees of hyponatremia of clinical importance. Carbamazepine-induced decreases in serum sodium appear dose-related and some evidence suggests that they may occur more readily in older patients. Thus, in any patient presenting with carbamazepine-induced confusion, serum sodium ought to be monitored in order to rule out hyponatremia and even the rare possibility of water intoxication. An occasional serum sodium when one is monitoring complete blood counts or carbamazepine levels may thus be clinically prudent, and serum electrolytes should be part of the initial base-line workup prior to starting medications, although it is not absolutely mandatory.

The incidence of carbamazepine-induced rash is reported between 10 and 15% in psychiatric populations, in contrast to just a few percent in most neurological studies. It is unclear whether this represents a true increased potential for carbamazepine-induced allergy in psychiatric compared with neurological populations or to some other variable, including closer assessment of dermatological side effects in the use of an unapproved agent. Nonetheless, attention to this issue is of some concern because of the potential for rashes to evolve into more serious exfoliative reactions or full-blown Stevens-Johnson syndrome. Given this possibility, it is perhaps prudent to discontinue carbamazepine upon appearance of a typical rash, which usually occurs between days 9 and 23 of treatment, although in a few instances, rashes can occur following more extended treatment. A small series of cases have been reported in which the carbamazepine rash has been successfully treated with prednisone (40 mg/day) upon restarting the drug without reemergence of the rash. In the neurological cases this has been reserved for patients without evidence of systemic toxicity and in patients who are otherwise refractory to other treatments. Thus, in psychiatric patients in the face of such a rash, it might be prudent to attempt other treatment regimes before returning to a clinical trial of carbamazepine with steroid cotreatment for suppression of the rash.

As with many other anticonvulsants, isolated cases of severe hepatitis have been reported with carbamazepine. On biopsy, these show lesions that appear toxic-metabolic or inflammatory. Benign increases in liver function tests are reported in a moderate percentage of patients in many studies, in most instances not requiring drug discontinuation.

Rare allergic syndromes have been reported such as pulmonitis with or without lymphadenopathy.

Carbamazepine appears to have a generally benign effect on cardiac function, although it clearly can decrease atrioventricular conduction times and should be used with great caution in any patient demonstrating varying degrees of heart block. In animals, carbamazepine has been demonstrated to reverse digitalis- and anoxia-induced ventricular tachycardias.

Management of the bipolar patient who wishes to become pregnant presents unique medical difficulties in the face of evidence that lithium carbonate can cause significant cardiac abnormalities (Ebstein's anomaly), particularly when administered during the first trimester of pregnancy. Therefore, rather than exposing patients intending to become pregnant to this small, but potentially very real, catastrophic consequence of lithium therapy, alternatives should be explored. Although no drug can be considered safe when administered during pregnancy, because of a variety of serious methodological difficulties and flaws in existing studies and data-gathering techniques, preliminary data suggest that carbamazepine, in contrast to several other agents, is not associated with specific syndromes of congenital anomalies. For example, phenytoin and the barbiturates have been associated with the fetal hydantoin syndrome. Valproate has been associated with spina bifida.

In contrast, carbamazepine has been extensively studied in animal model systems without a significant increase in anomalies over base-line, except when used in combination with valproate. Many epileptic patients treated with carbamazepine have been monitored for the incidence of anomalies, and no excess over base line has been established in these clinical studies. A recent report suggests that carbamazepine treatment might be associated with initially slightly decreased head size, body weight, and body length, but this rapidly normalized in the first months of life.

Thus, it would appear that carbamazepine, and possibly clonazepam, may be alternative agents to lithium in the management of the bipolar patient wishing to become pregnant. However, as discussed below, one cannot assume that a patient who is responsive to lithium carbonate will also respond to carbamazepine. In fact, the existing literature suggests that there may be differential subgroups of patients responsive to one or another agent, with a relatively small group overlapping. Given this circumstance, it might be wise to add carbamazepine to the otherwise well-maintained bipolar patient and then slowly taper lithium carbonate. This strategy is all the more advisable in light of recent evidence that discontinuation of lithium can be associated with withdrawal-emergent episodes.

A series of studies shows that severe episodes of mania and depression can occur in the several weeks immediately following lithium discontinuation with placebo, findings not observed with blind continuation treatment. Angst (1988, personal communication) reported that 80% of his patients who discontinue lithium have relapses. In some studies, lithium-induced withdrawal episodes appear to be occurring in spite of concomitant neuroleptic treatment, particularly in schizoaffective patients. Instability of the illness course during lithium treatment appeared to be a particularly bad prognostic sign for lithium withdrawal episodes, although in some instances withdrawal-emergent episodes were reported even in patients who had been well maintained for long periods of time without a recurrence.

Thus, when lithium discontinuation is being considered, it would appear most conservative to initiate a very slow tapering of the drug. If episodes emerge in spite of carbamazepine cotreatment, perhaps clonazepam rather than valproate could be considered as an alternative in the women wishing to become pregnant. Obviously, the strategy of searching for alternatives to lithium is based on the appropriate assessment with life-chart techniques (see Fig. 7-13), documenting on the basis of the prior course of illness that pharmacotherapy is in fact needed during the interval when the patient is attempting to become pregnant. In some bipolar patients, rather long well intervals may occur between expected episodes, and it may be possible for some patients to be maintained in a medication-free state. Even in this instance, extremely slow tapering of lithium over some weeks to months is again recommended.

Carbamazepine Prophylaxis

Both controlled and uncontrolled studies indicate that carbamazepine may play an important role in long-term prophylaxis of manic and depressive episodes. The efficacy of this anticonvulsant has been demonstrated in a small study against placebo and in two larger studies that were double-blind and randomized against lithium. Moreover, in lithium refractory patients, the addition of carbamazepine to existing ineffective regimes has led to substantial clinical improvement compared with base-line when patients are studied in a mirror image design. Overall, good to excellent responses to carbamazepine prophylaxis, either alone or in combination with lithium, have been reported in 252 of 373 patients (67%).

Given the general proclivity for the course of manic-depressive illness to deteriorate over time, with increasing severity and/or frequency of cycling, the impact of the addition of carbamazepine can be substantial. Figure 7-8 illustrates several cases from the NIMH who experienced repeated episodes of mania (graphed above the line) and depression (below the line) prior to the initiation of carbamazepine treatment (left side of dotted line). Following the addition of carbamazepine (right side) alone or as an adjunct to previously ineffective medication, a notable decrease in the frequency and severity of episodes is observed. However, in several instances, episodes began to reemerge after variable periods of extended clinical improvement.

A series of 24 patients who were preselected for good acute responses to carbamazepine at NIMH and then were maintained on carbamazepine prophylaxis in the community were followed. Patients were followed for an average of 4 years (range, 1–10 years). As illustrated in Fig. 7-9, carbamazepine made a substantial impact on the course of illness. In the 4 years prior to initiation of carbamazepine treatment, the illness appeared to be demonstrating an accelerating course with increasing severity as assessed by the illness index. The illness index is comprised by multiplying the duration of an episode times its severity with a moderate level of incapacity representing 0.5 and a severe level (complete incapacity or hospitalization) representing 1.0. Thus, 22 on the scale would represent 22 weeks of complete incapacitation or 44 weeks of moderate illness. In the group as a whole, carbamazepine substantially decreased the illness index over the years of follow-up. However, as illustrated in Fig. 7-10, this effect was composed of patients who maintained a stable degree of clinical improvement (top) and the other half of the patients who showed a pattern of marked improvement initially, but some escape from prophylaxis or reemergence of episodes in the 2nd or 3rd year of carbamazepine treatment as illustrated at the bottom of the figure.

The reasons for this apparent loss of efficacy were not obvious and

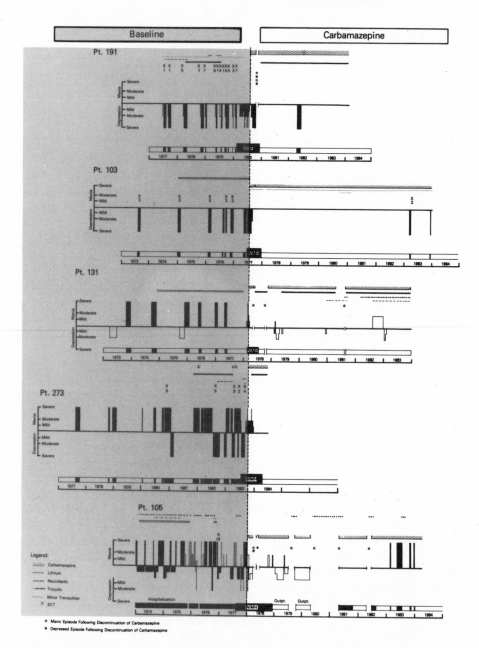

FIG. 7-8. Prophylactic efficacy of carbamazepine.

there were no systematic clinical markers of the stable group versus the escape group other than the escape group's having a more rapid acceleration in numbers of episodes in the 4 years prior to initiation of treatment compared with the stable group, which showed a level, and consistently

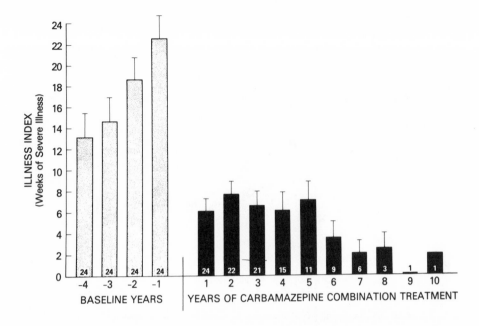

FIG. 7-9. Carbamazepine prophylaxis of primary affective illness (illness index represents duration of illness times its severity: 0.25 = mild; 0.05 = moderate; 1.0 = severe).

high, number of episodes prior to treatment initiation. These data are consistent with others in the literature which suggests that a proportion of patients showing a good acute or initial prophylactic response may begin to demonstrate relapses with chronic treatment.

One possible mechanism for this effect is the development of tolerance. This has not been systematically reported with carbamazepine in the treatment of seizures, although it is a recognized hazard in the long-term treatment of trigeminal neuralgia. Ways of avoiding this problem have not been systematically studied and it is now not clear whether increased dosages would be sufficient to restore therapeutic efficacy. In a preclinical model, Weiss and Post examined the development of tolerance to the anticonvulsant effects of carbamazepine and discovered that the tolerance is conditional. That is, if animals were repeatedly given carbamazepine prior to an amygdala-kindled seizure, they eventually began to demonstrate the reemergence of seizures (loss of efficacy). However, if the control group received carbamazepine after each kindled seizure, tolerance was not evident when the animals were given carbamazepine as a pretreatment. Therefore, it would appear that learning or conditioning mechanisms are involved.

This view is consistent with the observation that once tolerance has developed to carbamazepine's effects on amygdala-kindled seizures, a pe-

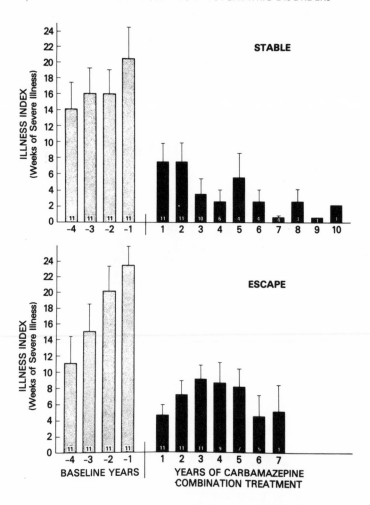

FIG. 7-10. Persistence of carbamazepine prophylaxis (illness index represents duration of illness times severity).

riod of treatment with carbamazepine after (but not before) the seizure has occurred or a period of seizures without any drug treatment is sufficient to reverse the tolerance phenomenon. Merely waiting an extended period of time (up to 3 weeks) or continuing carbamazepine treatment in the absence of kindled seizures is not sufficient to reverse the conditioned tolerance. In this preclinical model, increasing the dose of carbamazepine did not decrease the rate of tolerance development; neither did a regimen of alternating carbamazepine treatment with diazepam, even though there was no cross-tolerance between the two drugs. However, the one manipulation that appeared to slow the development of tolerance was the administration of carbamazepine (orally) at times other than immediately prior to an amygdala-kindled seizure. Viewed from the prospective of conditioned tolerance, this may have lessened the association between drug and seizure state. Given the evidence that a period of administering carbamazepine after seizures or the occurrence of seizures without medications did reverse the conditioned tolerance, it is wondered whether a period of time off of carbamazepine in people showing escape from its therapeutic efficacy in bipolar illness might also be sufficient to renew therapeutic efficacy. This speculative approach based on the preclinical model deserves to be tested in clinical trials and is obviously only a hypothetical approach to be explored and is not yet ready for routine clinical practice. However, it does illustrate the possible utility of animal models in helping to develop and direct clinical strategies. Fawcett (1988, personal communication) has reported his observations that a similar phenomenon can develop with the MAOIs and that patients who are initially responsive to the drug begin to develop breakthrough depressions. Consistent with the above concepts, Fawcett and Kravitz reported that a time off MAOIs is sufficient to reestablish therapeutic efficacy.

Until the mechanism is definitively elucidated and ways of circumventing potential tolerance development are found, it is perhaps most judicious for the physician to attempt either adjunctive or alternative treatments for the patient initially showing a good response. A series of alternative anticonvulsant strategies are reviewed below.

Potentiating carbamazepine treatment with other agents certainly deserves consideration. It has been observed that the addition of lithium to carbamazepine is helpful in potentiating its acute antidepressant and acute antimanic effectiveness; in addition we have observed a similar phenomenon with the addition of lithium to carbamazepine in the inadequate responder to prophylaxis. If patients are already on the lithium-carbamazepine combination and demonstrating escape, one might explore the utility of thyroid potentiation for prophylaxis. This strategy has a long tradition starting with the work of Gjessing (1975) in periodic catatonia and proceeding through the series of case reports and clinical vignettes from several investigative groups. Initially, good responses have been observed using a subgroup with thyroid alone, but more recent observations suggest the utility of adding thyroid to existing treatments. It has been observed that a recapturing of clinical response in this fashion occurs in a small series of patients. In addition, it has been noted that the addition of thyroid treatment to only partially effective combination treatment with lithium, carbamazepine, and valproate resulted in a complete remission in an ultrarapidly cycling patient who had been ill for 30 years. It will be important to follow closely the literature on thyroid potentiation for long-term prophylaxis in order to assess the degree of efficacy, possible mechanisms, and importance of T_3 versus T_4 at either replacement or hypermetabolic doses. Until these data are expanded, it is suggested that suppressive doses of T_3 or T_4 be administered. The induction of hyperthyroidism with hypermetabolic doses can have substantial medical complications particularly in older patients.

Adjunctive treatment with other nonanticonvulsant agents has just begun to be explored. Very preliminary data suggest that folate may improve long-term lithium prophylaxis compared with a placebo. Other vitamin manipulations remain to be explored, as does the treatment with catecholamine and indolamine precursors. Some data suggest the addition of the serotonin precursors L-tryptophan or 5-hydroxytryptophan (5-HTP) may serve an adjunctive role in long-term prophylaxis. The role of calcium channel blockers, which are not generally recognized as anticonvulsants (with the exception of nimodipine and flunarazine), also deserves further study as a possible adjunctive treatment. A series of case reports indicates the utility of verapamil in the treatment of acute mania, with limited promise for prophylaxis as well.

SODIUM VALPROATE

An analogue of valproate was first studied in a variety of psychiatric populations by Lambert and colleagues (1984) more than a decade ago. Clinically important acute and prophylactic effects in manic and depressive illness were observed. A clinical trial using a double-blind, on–off–on design also found the acute antimanic efficacy of valproate. In addition, a number of uncontrolled clinical trials from Germany, Poland, Japan, the United States, and South Africa all suggest that valproate may have positive effects in the treatment of manic-depressive illness on a prophylactic basis (Table 7-4). Several key points emerge from these data. It appears across these clinical trials that valproate has a considerably better profile on the acute and prophylactic treatment of manic compared with depressive episodes. Moreover, in most instances, valproate prophylaxis has been added to existing treatments such that its degree of clinical effi-

Table 7-4. Dipropylacetamide and Valproate Supplementation in Psychiatric Illness

Diagnosis	Good response/patients studied	Response (%)
Acute mania	30/56	54
Prophylaxis of mania/ depression	104/207	50
Schizoaffective	8/19	42
Acute depression	20/90	22
Schizophrenia	3/26	12

cacy alone, as opposed to in combination with lithium and/or neuroleptics, has not been adequately delineated. In some instances, when valproate has been given in combination with lithium carbonate and the lithium has been discontinued, relapses have been documented. Thus, in the face of this ambiguity regarding response to valproate alone, it would appear prudent to consider trials of valproate in combination with lithium in most instances.

If lithium discontinuation is to be attempted, one would recommend that this proceed in an extremely gradual fashion, as considerable evidence (mentioned above) now suggests that discontinuation of lithium may be associated with withdrawal-emergent episodes. However, whether or not a slow tapering of lithium is actually helpful in avoiding these episodes has not been adequately studied. In contrast to studies of a decade or more ago, more recent studies document the emergence of severe affective psychosis, most notably manias, when lithium is discontinued, in some studies even in the face of concomitant neuroleptic maintenance treatment. Preliminary markers for patients who show exacerbations on lithium discontinuation are those with schizoaffective illness, and an unstable clinical course prior to drug discontinuation. However, in some patients, lithium discontinuation has been reported to result in the emergence of episodes even after prolonged periods when patients have been maintained adequately in a well interval and an episode would not have been expected.

Thus, in the face of successful lithium prophylaxis either alone or in combination with anticonvulsants such as carbamazepine or valproic acid, the dangers of a clinical trial of lithium discontinuation should be given careful consideration before it is attempted. Perhaps the presence of compelling indicators of the need for discontinuation (such as the presence of severe or incapacitating side effects) are warranted before this action is attempted. In the face of problematic degrees of tremor, DI, psoriasis, or other typical lithium-induced side effects, perhaps the clinician should attempt dose reduction in a gradual fashion, rather than abrupt drug discontinuation. This might achieve the dual purpose of side-effect reduction as well as the assessment of whether decreases in lithium doses and blood levels are in fact associated with any signs of symptom recrudescence. If gradual reductions in lithium are not associated with the reemergence of symptoms, this might allow one to proceed cautiously toward discontinuation in the face of careful clinical monitoring.

Typical blood levels of valproic acid used in the treatment of manic-depressive patients have ranged between 50 and 100 μg/ml (i.e., the same range used in the treatment of patients with seizure disorders). These blood levels can often be achieved with doses in the range of 750–1,500 mg/day although sometimes higher doses are required. The clinical studies and case reports using valproate have been remarkable in terms of the absence of side effects in the psychiatric population. The most common side effects have been gastrointestinal complaints, tremor, increased appetite and weight gain, alopecia, and rashes.

In contrast to the occasional report of severe hepatitis and the very rare instances of fatal hepatic complications during valproate treatment of epileptics, these reactions have not been reported in psychiatric patients. In fact, recent reviews of the epilepsy literature on valproate suggest that these complications occur most commonly in patients under 2 years of age or in other patients treated with combination therapy. In spite of markedly increased use of valproate recently, the incidence of fatal hepatic reactions with the use of this compound appears to be small and not increasing. Initial assessment of hepatic function prior to the use of valproic acid and then periodic monitoring is recommended. Mild elevations of liver function tests are common, but the risk of potentially severe hepatic reactions would appear to be quite low in the adult affectively ill populations who would be receiving treatment with this agent. Thus, it would appear that valproic acid is not only the second best-studied anticonvulsant after carbamazepine, but also shows the second best profile of degree of clinical efficacy.

As is the case with carbamazepine, there are relatively few studies of the effects of valproate in depression, and the acute and prophylactic effects of valproate for the treatment of depression remain to be fully delineated in further clinical trials. Nonetheless, this agent is recommended as the second anticonvulsant (and third agent after lithium) to be considered in the prophylactic management of patients with bipolar disorder. Figure 7-11 illustrates a patient showing excellent response to the combination of valproate and lithium when he did not respond to carbamazepine. Patient 244 was a 46-year-old single male who showed a long history of repeated severe manic episodes requiring hospitalization in spite of lithium treatment. Five hospitalizations for mania occurred in the 4 years prior to NIMH admission. These episodes were completely incapacitating and this patient also demonstrated panic attacks during his manic episodes. During treatment with carbamazepine on a blind basis at NIMH, a manic episode emerged approximately "on schedule." Given this lack of efficacy of carbamazepine prophylaxis in this individual, valproic acid was added to lithium carbonate, which had previously been ineffective in preventing recurrent manic episodes. This patient has done well and has not had a recurrence of manic episodes requiring hospitalization for 5 years with valproate and lithium combination prophylaxis. This contrasts with multiple hospitalizations in the several years prior to NIMH hospitalization during treatment with lithium carbonate alone. Similar clinical responses to valproate and lithium combinations have been observed including one patient who is being treated with valproic acid alone with excellent results when carbamazepine in combination with lithium and MAOIs had not been previously effective.

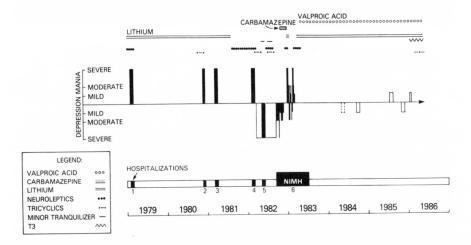

FIG. 7-11. Prophylactic response to valproic acid in a carbamazepine nonresponder (patient 244).

This case is presented in some detail in order to illustrate the point that a response to one anticonvulsant in a given individual may not be predictive of a response to another anticonvulsant. This has clearly been demonstrated in another patient who responded to carbamazepine remarkably, as illustrated in Fig. 7-12, but not to phenytoin or valproic acid. The converse has been illustrated in the above case presentation (see Fig. 7-11).

These cases suggest the utility of (1) a sequential series of trials of the anticonvulsants, particularly in the face of lack of efficacy of one anticonvulsant agent when used in combination with lithium carbonate, and (2) perhaps other adjunctive treatments, such as neuroleptics or nighttime benzodiazepines such as clonazepam for the nonresponsive patient.

Although systematic clinical trials have not been conducted comparing carbamazepine to valproate or even more importantly crossing over a large series of patients from one to another agent, sequential trials of the anticonvulsants would appear useful as a clinical strategy to be pursued in individual patients. Parenthetically, a clinician might be able to provide valuable empirical data for the literature if he were able to systematically cross over patients from one to another of these agents, even in an open clinical design. The delineation of potential clinical and biological markers of response to one or another of these anticonvulsants in affectively ill patients would obviously be of great clinical and theoretical interest.

It is clear that carbamazepine and valproate have very different anticonvulsant profiles. In particular, carbamazepine has been reported to exacerbate generalized absence seizures in some patients, whereas valproic acid clearly has a positive clinical profile on this seizure type, as well

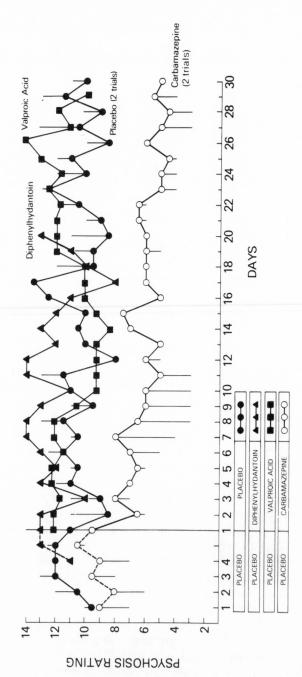

FIG. 7-12. Carbamazepine but not diphenylhydantoin or valproic acid decreases manic psychosis in a patient with manic-depressive illness. Drug administration and nurse's rating were achieved on a double-blind basis.

as on a variety of others. It is of some interest that among the anticonvulsants, carbamazepine and valproic acid are the first and second agents in the rank order of potency in inhibiting amygdala-kindled seizures compared with those kindled from the cerebral cortex. This measure provides an indirect assessment of the ability to stabilize limbic seizures; it may not be coincidental that these two drugs show the greatest degree of clinical promise in the treatment of manic-depressive illness.

However, there is very little direct evidence to support the view that the efficacy of carbamazepine (or valproate) is related to its ability to stabilize limbic system excitability. The degree of clinical response to carbamazepine is not related to the presence of EEG abnormalities in psychiatric patients, reports of psychosensory symptoms, degree of clinical response to procaine or associated EEG activation of fast activity over the temporal lobes, or other potential markers of limbic excitability that can be measured in affectively ill patients. In a similar vein, there is essentially no data linking the ability of valproate to stabilize temporal lobe or limbic substrates to its positive effects in manic-depressive illness. Although there was an initial report that patients with abnormal EEGs responded better to valproate treatment for their manic-depressive illness, this was not confirmed in an extension of that clinical trial. Given this lack of clinical and biological markers for response to anticonvulsants, again it is recommended that sequential clinical trials be employed for the refractory bipolar patient.

CLONAZEPAM AND RELATED ANTICONVULSANT BENZODIAZEPINES

Clonazepam is a benzodiazepine anticonvulsant with exclusive actions at the central-type benzodiazepine receptor which is linked to a γ-amino butyric acid (GABA)-receptor that modulates a chloride ion channel. GABA appears to be the major inhibitory neurotransmitter in the brain. Benzodiazepines such as diazepam and clonazepam facilitate GABA-mediated inhibition resulting in increases in chloride intercellularly which stabilizes cell membranes. The muscle relaxant, antianxiety, and anticonvulsant effects of the benzodiazepines, thus, are all thought to be mediated by *agonist* actions at this receptor site. Recently, a class of compounds called *inverse agonists* has been discovered that appears to have opposite biochemical and physiological effects. These inverse agonists, particularly the betacarboline class, exert anxiogenic and proconvulsant effects. These substances have been used to model anxiety in animal laboratory studies and in two instances, an inverse agonist administered to humans produced severe anxiety reactions that were benzodiazepine-agonist reversible.

Another class of compounds that is essentially neutral and blocks the effects of both agonists and inverse agonists at the benzodiazepine receptor has also been uncovered. These compounds include Ro15-1788 and CGS-8216, and have been useful in elucidating mechanisms of action of drugs that are specifically mediated through the benzodiazepine receptor. For example, Ro15-1788 reverses the anticonvulsant effects of diazepam on amygdala-kindled seizures, although it is without effect on carbamazepine's anticonvulsant effects. Conversely, a ligand which acts at the so-called peripheral-type benzodiazepine receptor Ro5-4864 reverses the anticonvulsant effects of carbamazepine, but does not affect those of diazepam. Taken together, these data suggest that the anticonvulsant effects of the benzodiazepines are mediated through the central-type benzodiazepine receptor, whereas those of carbamazepine are mediated through the so-called peripheral-type receptor. Although intravenous diazepam is a potent anticonvulsant in man, when it is orally administered, diazepam is ineffective as an anticonvulsant. In contrast, clonazepam, alprazolam, and lorazepam all appear to exert anticonvulsant properties when administered orally. As such, these later agents appear to possess a range of clinical efficacy that makes them of potential use in the treatment of manic-depressive illness.

It is clear that alprazolam and clonazepam have excellent antipanic properties, although they may have differential antimanic and (limited) antidepressant effects (see below). Clonazepam has been used in the treatment of complex partial and generalized absence seizures. Tolerance to its anticonvulsant effects has been reported in preclinical models as well as in patients. There is also some evidence that tolerance can develop to the antipanic effects of clonazepam and alprazolam. A study of the long-term use of clonazepam in the treatment of manic-depressive illness suggests the development of tolerance in approximately one-third of patients. Given this possibility as well as the moderate sedating properties of clonazepam, this drug might have an unique and important use in potentiating the antimanic effects of other agents, particularly when used as a nighttime sedative, rather than as a first-line treatment.

It is thus recommended that clonazepam be used for manic breakthroughs and for the early appearance of sleep loss in a patient who is being prophylactically treated with other agents. Use of clonazepam in this fashion may have advantages over the use of neuroleptics for this indication, as clonazepam is devoid of extrapyramidal side effects and its use may also help avoid the possibility of continuing longer-term maintenance treatment with neuroleptics and the subsequent risk of tardive dyskinesia.

While the acute manic efficacy of clonazepam has not been extensively studied, initial double-blind reports suggest that it has an antimanic efficacy comparable with that of lithium carbonate. Recent anecdotal reports also attest to its mood-stabilizing properties in severe manic and schizoaffective states. The ability of clonazepam to acutely treat or prevent depressive recurrences has not been systematically investigated except in one clinical trial from Japan suggesting prophylactic effectiveness against both manic and depressive episodes (Kishimoto and Okuma, 1988, personal communication).

Clearly, further work is necessary to delineate the spectrum of clinical efficacy of this anticonvulsant as well as the degree of the problem with tolerance development. Because there is some evidence for the initial loss of efficacy with the anticonvulsant carbamazepine (which has not been associated with the development of tolerance in most animal models and clinical antiepileptic studies), one might expect even more substantial problems with clonazepam which has been closely linked to tolerance development. Moreover, there are isolated reports of the precipitation of depressive episodes in panic patients treated with benzodiazepine anticonvulsants, further raising the question whether this might not also occur in a subgroup of affectively ill patients. Carbamazepine-related induction of depression does not appear to be a general problem in affective disorder patients, although in patients with borderline personality disorder, several instances have been reported in which patients' base line mood instability has been converted to a more endogenomorphic and protracted depression.

Because some patients find clonazepam highly sedating, initial doses of 0.5–1 mg are recommended. Antimanic effects occur in most patients in the range of 1–4 mg/day. Higher doses may be attempted, but these are likely to be associated with greater degrees of sedation and theoretically a more rapid induction of tolerance. Clonazepam has the advantage of being a non-neuroleptic antimanic agent which is usually well tolerated, is safe in overdose, and not only does not produce extrapyramidal side effects, but has been used in the treatment of some extrapyramidal motor disorders, including akathisia with some success.

Alprazolam also appears to exert anticonvulsant effects through the central-type benzodiazepine receptor, although preliminary evidence suggests that it may also have indirect interactions with the peripheral-type benzodiazepine site. In doses of 1–4 mg/day, alprazolam appears to exert excellent antipanic effects. The onset of antipanic efficacy appears faster than that achieved by traditional agents including tricyclic antidepressants and MAOIs. However, in controlled clinical trials, this advantage appears to be lost by the third or fourth week of treatment when the conventional agents catch up or exceed alprazolam in their degree of efficacy.

This has led some clinicians to initiate antipanic treatment with a tricyclic or a MAOI in conjunction with cotreatment with alprazolam in order to help the panic-prone patient through the initial several weeks of treatment. This appears also to be useful in light of the fact that in some instances, panic-prone patients are sensitive to even initial low doses of tricyclics at the beginning of therapy. Many patients appear to show persistent antipanic effects during long-term treatment with alprazolam without dose increases. However, a subgroup of patients appears to demonstrate a loss of efficacy and/or require dose increases to maintain a degree of antipanic control. This phenomenon, taken in conjunction with the reports of the extreme difficulty in a subgroup of patients with even slow tapering of alprazolam withdrawal, leads to the suggestion that alprazolam should be reserved for more selected use in the panic-prone patient. This might be as an initial adjunct (as described) or for patients who do not otherwise respond to tricyclic antidepressants, the MAOIs, or the selective serotonin reuptake blockers which also appear to show an important profile as antipanic as well as antidepressant agents.

In addition, there is some cause for concern regarding the use of alprazolam in bipolar patients. Like the tricyclic antidepressants, alprazolam has been reported to be associated with the precipitation of mania in bipolar patients. This phenomenon has also been reported in some panic patients without a prior history of mania as well. Similar reports have not been forthcoming with benzodiazepine clonazepam. Thus, it would appear that some component of alprazolam's triazolo structure may be associated with additional properties which, like the tricyclic antidepressants, make it less desirable in the treatment of bipolar patients.

ACETAZOLAMIDE

An initial report suggested that the carbonic anhydrase inhibitor anticonvulsant, acetazolamide (Diamox), may exert clinical efficacy in patients with a spectrum of atypical psychoses (Inoue et al., 1984). In particular, those with dreamy confusional states and episodes recurrently associated with the premenstrual phases or the puerperium might respond to this agent. It was noteworthy that in these instances, patients responded to acetazolamide when they had not responded to either lithium or carbamazepine. The degree of efficacy of this agent in more typical manic-depressive states and its utility in prophylaxis both remain to be further explored. However, given the apparent difference in responsivity to this anticonvulsant compared with carbamazepine, perhaps it deserves a clinical trial low on the rank order of priorities in the otherwise refractory bipolar patient. In the Japanese studies, the doses ranged from 500 to 1,000 mg/day.

PHENYTOIN

Phenytoin (Dilantin) remains a mystery drug in relationship to its efficacy in manic-depressive patients. It appears to have an anticonvulsant profile very similar to that of carbamazepine in the treatment of major motor and partial seizures. However, it is substantially less effective in animal models of limbic epilepsy, such as that observed with amygdala kindling. Like carbamazepine, it also appears effective in a subgroup of patients with trigeminal neuralgia. Given this convergence of clincial actions comparable with that of carbamazepine and the ability of both agents to stabilize sodium channel flux (particularly under conditions of depolarization and fast firing), common antimanic effects might be expected.

However, clinical reports with phenytoin are mixed at best. Initial open studies suggested the utility of phenytoin in manic and schizoaffective states, although a subsequent study failed to demonstrate efficacy. The issue would appear to merit careful reexamination using double-blind clinical trials, but as yet none are available. In five manic-depressive patients not responsive to carbamazepine, Post and colleagues (1987) have observed no patient responding to phenytoin administered on a blind basis. Perhaps a higher rate of response would be observed in a population not preselected for carbamazepine nonresponse. Nonetheless, in the absence of positive data from controlled studies or even recent anecdotal reports, it would appear that this agent should be reserved for clinical trials in the patient who is unable to tolerate or does not respond to carbamazepine or any of the other anticonvulsants, rather than a first-line treatment alternative.

Development of systematic comparative data of the antimanic efficacy of phenytoin compared to carbamazepine would be of clinical as well as theoretical interest. If the two had equal antimanic efficacy, common mechanisms such as sodium channel stabilization might be implicated. If carbamazepine clearly emerged as superior, unique effects of this compound might be given higher consideration as related to its antimanic properties. This might include the ability of carbamazepine to increase plasma tryptophan, act as an adenosine receptor antagonist, increase synaptic dopamine, inhibit a variety of adenylate cyclases, and decrease somatostatin. It is of interest that the antimanic agents, lithium, carbamazepine, valproate, propranolol, and progabide, all decrease GABA turnover.

γ-AMINOBUTYRIC ACID AGONISTS

GABA agonists, which have recently been demonstrated to possess anticonvulsant effectiveness in animal models and in the clinic, have been suggested as potential antidepressant agents. In a series of open and double-blind clinical trials, efficacy in mild-to-moderate depression, and responses comparable with those seen with traditional tricyclic antidepressants have been observed. More systematic studies of their efficacy in mania as well as in prophylaxis need to be performed before these agents can be recommended in the treatment of bipolar patients. Nonetheless, they represent a novel and promising alternative category of agents that deserve further study among the anticonvulsant class.

A subclass of GABA-active agents is thought to act on a selective $GABA_B$ receptor or one that responds preferentially to the agonist baclofen. Although baclofen has been useful in the treatment of trigeminal neuralgia, it does not appear to have potent anticonvulsant effects in most animal models (although it will decrease hippocampal excitability in selected regions of this structure). Preliminary clinical trials with a $GABA_B$ agonist, L-baclofen, have not yielded promising results in depressed patients to date, however. These findings are of potential theoretical interest in light of the reports from the laboratory of Lloyd (1986) that chronic but not acute administration of all known antidepressant modalities (tricyclics, MAOIs, ECT) upregulate $GABA_B$ receptors in the frontal cortex of experimental animals. Observations of Terrence et al. (1983) indicate that the $GABA_B$ properties of carbamazepine may be responsible for its clinical efficacy in the treatment of trigeminal neuralgia whereas studies by Weiss and Post (unpublished) indicate that $GABA_B$ effects are not related to the anticonvulsant effects of carbamazepine on amygdala-kindled seizures. Whether direct treatment with the $GABA_B$ agonist, L-baclofen would have a role in the manic-depressive disorder remains doubtful, suggesting that $GABA_B$ effects of carbamazepine may be related to its efficacy in trigeminal neuralgia, but not epilepsy or affective illness.

CALCIUM CHANNEL BLOCKERS

A small series of double-blind clinical trials and clinical reports suggest that the calcium channel blockers such as verapamil may exert antimanic effects. Although verapamil is not a potent anticonvulsant, two other calcium channel blockers, nimodipine and flunarizine, are anticonvulsants and have been reported effective in either animal models or in preliminary clinical trials (flunarizine). The profile of calcium channel blockers in long-term efficacy remains to be delineated, but a clinical trial of these compounds would appear indicated in the otherwise refractory bipolar patient. Typical doses of verapamil have ranged from 240 to 480 mg/day.

GRAPHIC DEPICTION OF LIFE COURSE OF ILLNESS

An adequate understanding and graphic depiction of the recurrent nature of the affective disorders is critical to their successful treatment. In approaching the pharmacotherapy of this serious and potentially life-threatening medical illness, attention should be paid to the detailing of the prior course of illness retrospectively, as well as graphing mood fluctuations prospectively. In this fashion, the need for acute pharmacological interventions can be integrated with the longitudinal course of the illness. In some cases tricyclics and MAOIs may be required in the bipolar patient to treat acute depressive episodes. However, this prescription may be at the cost of precipitating manic episodes or inducing more rapid cycling of the illness. Assessment with life-chart methodology helps convey and demonstrate the longitudinal course of the illness which provides a backdrop for whatever acute pharmacotherapeutic interventions are being attempted. Moreover, the adequacy of previous pharmacotherapy and the evaluation of partial responses can be more accurately assessed using this technique. The patient's participation is obviously critical in this process which may have a secondary positive effect of increasing the therapeutic alliance and patient compliance with medical and pharmacological recommendations. With graphic depiction of episodes, the illness' relationship to seasonal patterns, life events, and other environmental impacts is often more readily elucidated than when one only takes a verbal history. In this fashion, periods of increased vulnerability can be assessed and adequate acute and prophylactic interventions at these time frames can be considered.

Figure 7-13 presents a scheme for constructing such a life chart. Severity of manic and depressive episodes are based on three degrees of functional impairment: mild, moderate, or severe. In the mild category, the patient is aware of distinct mood changes different from his normal usual self, but function is not notably impaired. In the moderate category, symptoms meet the *Diagnostic and Statistical Manual of Mental Disorders* (DSM-III) criteria and in addition are associated with moderate to substantial functional impairment in the patient's ability to perform his usual professional or social activities but only with great effort. In the severe category, the patient is functionally incapacitated and/or hospitalized (which can be indicated by a shading of the episodes). Medications can be coded above these episodes and life events and important comments can be included below the episode line. Patients should be encouraged to keep a calendar based on a 100-mm line mood scale, 0 being most depressed or worst ever, 50 being usual self, and 100 being highest or most manic ever. This scale can then be integrated with a functional impairment scale and life charting can proceed in a prospective fashion. In this way adequate base lines can be established for the assessment of the efficacy of recommended treatments.

The importance of this methodology for patients who are being treated with anticonvulsants as second-line strategies (for those who do not do well on lithium carbonate or who are unable to tolerate its side effects) is emphasized. In these instances patients tend to have multiple episodes (Fig. 7-14), experience pharmacological precipitation of manic episodes with tricyclics or MAOIs, and have a number of risk factors for relative nonresponse to pharmacotherapy such as rapid cycling, associated personality disorders, drug or alcohol abuse, and a pattern of episodes marked by depressions immediately followed by manias (rather than the converse, i.e., mania followed by a depression, which often responds well to lith-

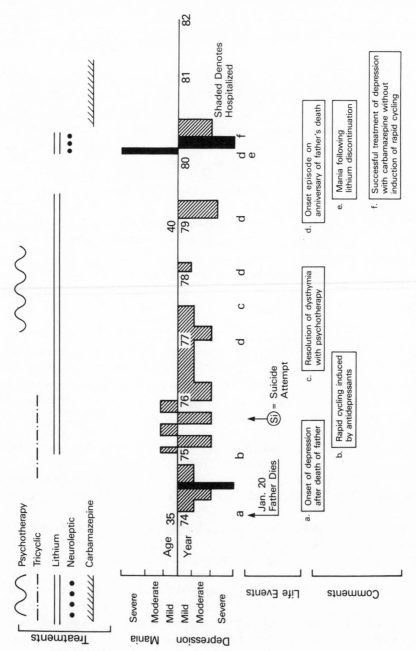

FIG. 7-13. Graphing the course of affective illness. This is a prototype of a life chart.

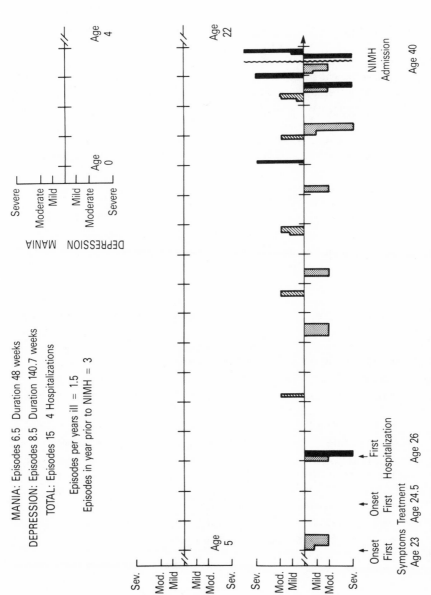

FIG. 7-14. Median course of affective illness in 82 bipolar manic-depressive patients.

ium). Thus, accurate record keeping and tracking of the illness might be parallel to accurate assessment of the amount of glucose being spilled in the urine of an unstable diabetic or accurate and ongoing assessment of the location and size of metastases in the patient with a primary malignancy. It is only with precise assessment of these illness-monitoring measures that one can establish the adequacy of the medical intervention.

Although this discussion has highlighted and focused on a primary role for pharmacological interventions acutely and prophylactically in manic-depressive illness, it is important to reemphasize the critical need for psychological support, psychotherapy, and family and social support systems. There is increasing evidence for the efficacy of cognitive and interpersonal therapies in the treatment of acute depressive episodes. Increased psychological support may not only aid in facilitating compliance with pharmacotherapy, it may have a positive interaction with pharmacotherapy in treatment of the patient with recurrent affective illness. Regular visits to monitor drug blood levels, potential side effects, and the progress of treatment (in conjunction with supportive psychotherapy), may further assist in the therapeutic alliance, drug compliance, and may be a very positive factor in the remoralization process and in the avoidance of suicide. There are increasing data that in patients with recurrent affective disorders, the risk of suicide, often prominent early in the illness after an initial episode, can also increase with the duration of the illness. Thus, helping to educate the patient and his family about the availability of many pharmacological alternatives (now including a range of anticonvulsants), the time required to make adequate assessments of their acute and prophylactic efficacy (often considerable), and a range of other positive psychological and psychosocial interventions may be critical in helping the patient through difficult periods of affective crisis that often occur with manic or depressive recurrences.

The truly skilled pharmacotherapist of the affective disorders should be able to prescribe and incorporate a wide variety of pharmacotherapeutic and psychotherapeutic treatment modalities to maximum advantage in attempting to give optimal assistance to his patients suffering from the medical, psychologically demoralizing, and stigmatizing effects of recurrent manic and depressive episodes. Adequate use of the anticonvulsants and other recently documented treatments may make as great or greater an impact on the lives of patients with recurrent affective disorders as on those with seizure disorders.

REFERENCES AND SUGGESTED READING

Ballenger JC, Post RM. Carbamazepine (Tegretol) in manic-depressive illness: a new treatment. *Am J Psychiatry* 1980;137:782–790.
Chouinard G, Young SN, Annable L. Antimanic effect of clonazepam. *Biol Psychiatry* 1983;18:451–466.

Dalby MA. Antiepileptic and psychotropic effect of carbamazepine (Tegretol) in the treatment of psychomotor epilepsy. *Epilepsia* 1971;12:325–334.

De Montigny C, Grunberg F, Mayer A, Deschenes JP. Lithium induces rapid relief of depression in tricyclic antidepressant drug nonresponders. *Br J Psychiatry* 1981;138:252–256.

Emrich HM, von Zerssen D, Kissling W, Moller HJ, Windorfer A. Effect of sodium valproate in mania. The GABA-hypothesis of affective disorders. *Arch Psychiatr Nervenkr* 1980;229:1–16.

Fawcett J, Kravitz DO. The long-term management of bipolar disorders with lithium, carbamazepine, and antidepressants: clinical experience with 90 cases. *J Clin Psychiatry* 1985;46:58–60.

Gallicchio VS, Hulette BC. In vitro effect of lithium on carbamazepine-induced inhibition of murine and human bone marrow derived granulocyte-macrophage and megakaryocyte progenitor stem cells. *Exp Biol Med* (in press).

Gjessing LR. Academic address: a review of periodic catatonia. *Biol Psychiatry* 1975;8:23–45.

Inoue H, Hazama H, Hamazoe K, et al. Antipsychotic and prophylactic effects of acetazolamide (Diamox) on atypical psychosis. *Folia Psychiatr Neurol Jpn* 1984;38:425–436.

Joffe RT, Post RM, Roy-Byrne PP, Uhde TW. Hematological effects of carbamazepine in patients with affective illness. *Am J Psychiatry* 1985;142:1196–1199.

Joffe RT, Singer W. Thyroid hormone potentiation of antidepressants. *Biol Psychiatry* (in press).

Kishimoto A, Ogura C, Hazama H, Inoue K. Long-term prophylactic effects of carbamazepine in affective disorder. *Br J Psychiatry* 1983;143:327–331.

Kramlinger KG, Post RM. The addition of lithium carbonate to carbamazepine: antidepressant efficacy in treatment-resistant depression. *Arch Gen Psychiatry* (in press).

Lambert PA. Acute and prophylactic therapies of patients with affective disorders using valpromide (dipropylacetamide). In: Emrich HM, Okuma T, Muller AA (eds). *Anticonvulsants in Affective Disorders.* Amesterdam: Excerpta Medica, 1984:33–44.

Lloyd KG, Thuret EW, Pilc A. GABA and the mechanisms of action of antidepressant drugs. In: Bartholini G, Lloyd KG, Morselli PL, eds. *GABA and Mood Disorders: Animal and Clinical Studies.* New York: Raven Press, 1986:195–202. (L.E.R.S. Monograph Series; vol 4.)

McElroy SL, Keck PE, Jr, Pope HG, Jr. Sodium valproate: its use in primary psychiatric disorders. *J Clin Psychopharmacol* 1987;7:16–24.

Muller AA, Stoll K-D. Carbamazepine and oxcarbazepine in the treatment of manic syndromes: studies in Germany. In: Emrich HM, Okuma T, Muller AA, eds. *Anticonvulsants in Affective Disorders.* Amsterdam: Excerpta Medica, 1984:139–147.

Okuma T, Inanaga K, Otsuki S, Sarai K, Takahashi R, Hazama H, Mori A, Watanabe M. A preliminary double-blind study of the efficacy of carbamazepine in prophylaxis of manic-depressive illness. *Psychopharmacology* 1981;73:95–96.

Pellock JM. Carbamazepine side effects in children and adults. *Epilepsia* 1987;28:64S–70S.

Post RM. Effectiveness of carbamazepine in the treatment of bipolar affective disorders. In: McElroy S, Pope HG, eds. *Use of Anticonvulsants in Psychiatry: Recent Advances.* Clifton, NJ: Oxford Health Care, 1988:1–23.

Post RM, Ballenger JC, Uhde TW, Bunney WE, Jr. Efficacy of carbamazepine in manic-depressive illness: implications for underlying mechanisms. In: Post RM, Ballenger JC, eds. *Neurobiology of Mood Disorders.* Baltimore: Williams & Wilkins, 1984a:777–816.

Post RM, Berrettini W, Uhde TW, Kellner C. Selective response to the anticonvulsant carbamazepine in manic-depressive illness: a case study. *J Clin Psychopharmacol* 1984b;4:178–185.

Post RM, Rubinow DR, Ballenger JC. Conditioning and sensitization in the longitudinal course of affective illness. *Br J Psychiatry* 1986a;149:191–201.

Post RM, Uhde TW. Are the psychotropic effects of carbamazepine in manic-depressive illness mediated through the limbic system? *Psychiatr J Univ Ottawa* 1985;10:205–219.

Post RM, Uhde TW, Ballenger JC, Chatterji DC, Green RF, Bunney WE, Jr. Carbamazepine and its −10,11-epoxide metabolite in plasma and CSF: relationship to antidepressant response. *Arch Gen Psychiatry* 1983b;40:673–676.

Post RM, Uhde TW, Ballenger JC, Squillace KM. Prophylactic efficacy of carbamazepine in manic-depressive illness. *Am J Psychiatry* 1983a; 140:1602–1604.

Post RM, Uhde TW, Roy-Byrne PP, Joffe RT. Correlates of antimanic response to carbamazepine. *Psychiatr Res* 1987a;21:71–83.

Post RM, Uhde TW, Roy-Byrne RP, Joffe RT. Antidepressant effects of carbamazepine. *Am J Psychiatry* 1986b;143:29–34.

Post RM, Uhde TW, Rubinow DR, Huggins T. 1986c; Differential time course of antidepressant effects after sleep deprivation, ECT, and carbamazepine: clinical and theoretical implications. *Psychiatr Res* 1987b;22:11–19.

Silberman EK, Post RM, Nurnberger J, Theodore W, Boulenger JP. Transient sensory, cognitive, and affective phenomena in affective illness: a comparison with complex partial epilepsy. *Br J Psychiatry* 1985;146:81–89.

Terrence CF, Sax M, Fromm GH, Chang CH, Yoo CS. Effect of baclofen enantiomorphs on the spinal trigeminal nucleus and steric similarities of carbamazepine. *Pharmacology* 1983;27:85–94.

8

Anticonvulsants as Adjuncts to Neuroleptics in the Treatment of Schizoaffective and Schizophrenic Patients

Robert M. Post

PHARMACOLOGICAL BACKGROUND OF NEUROLEPTICS

The primary treatment modality for schizophrenic and related drug-induced psychoses remains the antipsychotic neuroleptics. With the exception of reserpine, which depletes the catecholamine dopamine, essentially all of the antipsychotic neuroleptic agents are thought to act by blocking dopamine receptors. There is a good correlation of their doses used clinically to treat psychotic patients and their ability to bind to dopamine receptors. In addition to the amphetamine model of schizophrenic psychosis, which postulates a causal role for excess dopamine, the therapeutic effects of the neuroleptics corresponding to their ability to block dopamine receptors form the cornerstone of the dopamine hypothesis of schizophrenia. The exquisite responsiveness of amphetamine and other stimulant-induced psychoses to the neuroleptics further supports such a view. Although an increase in dopamine in discrete areas of brain has been postulated, direct measurement of dopamine or its metabolite homovanillic acid in the brain or cerebrospinal fluid of schizophrenic patients has not consistently documented increased levels of these compounds. However, two recent studies have suggested a unilateral increase in dopamine in the left amygdala of schizophrenic patients studied at autopsy. More consistent are the autopsy findings of increased dopamine receptors, theoretically linked to an increased dopaminergic activity based on postsynaptic receptor sensitivity. However, a major problem with this hypothesis is that most schizophrenic patients have been treated with dopamine receptor-blocking agents and therefore would be expected to demonstrate long-term compensatory increases in dopamine receptors as

Table 8-1. Strategies for Neuroleptic Augmentation in Schizoaffective and Schizophrenic Illness

---

Lithium
Carbamazepine
Anticonvulsant benzodiazepines
  Clonazepam
  Alprazolam
Valproate
Acetazolamide[a]
Phenytoin
Propranolol
Calcium channel blockers
  (may worsen nonmanic psychosis)

---

[a]For atypical confusional psychosis with dreamy states occurring premenstrually or in puerperium.

a secondary effect of treatment rather than as a primary effect of their illness.

Adjunctive treatments to the neuroleptics (Table 8-1) are required for a variety of reasons. Although there is an overwhelming demonstration of the efficacy of neuroleptics compared with other compounds or placebos in the acute and prophylactic treatment of schizophrenic patients, many patients do not respond completely or adequately. Often, the positive symptoms of schizophrenic hallucinations and delusions improve to a relatively greater degree than the negative symptoms such as thought disorder, paralysis of will, withdrawal, and autism.

Furthermore, the neuroleptic agents have a series of inherent liabilities. With the exception of clozapine, they are all capable of producing acute parkinsonian and related extrapyramidal side effects such as dystonia (Table 8-2). These often require management with anticholinergic agents. Even more problematic is the emergence of tardive dyskinesia with long-term use of neuroleptics. In some instances, this syndrome can be cosmetically disfiguring and medically disabling, and does not respond readily to any therapeutic modality available to date. Various studies have suggested that the dose and duration of neuroleptic treatment, as well as female sex, diagnosis of affective illness, and possibly even the number of intervals off of medication, could all be risk factors for the development of this potentially disabling syndrome (Table 8-3). There is some evidence, however, that dyskinetic dysfunctional motor phenomena similar to tardive dyskinesia were observed in psychotic patients in the prepsychopharmacological era. Thus, the contribution of disordered chemical substrates related to the primary psychiatric disorder versus the effects of the neu-

Table 8-2. Extrapyramidal Side Effects of Neuroleptics
(Except Clozapine)

	Anticholinergic reversible
Acute treatment	
Parkinsonism	+ +
Tremor	+
Dystonia	+ +
Oculogyral crisis	+ +
Akathisia	±
Neuroleptic malignant syndrome	−
Chronic treatment	
Parkinsonism (late)	+ + +[a]
Akathisia	±
Tardive dyskinesia	−
Tardive dystonia	−
(Neuroleptic malignant syndrome)	−
Irreversible neurotoxicity with lithium	−
(Haloperidol at higher risk?)	

[a]? Lesser need for anticholinergics with chronic treatment.

Table 8-3. Possible Risk Factors for Tardive Dyskinesia

Age
Female sex
Depressive or bipolar affective illness
Neurological dysfunction
High dose or cumulative dose
Length of treatment (nonlinear; probably threshold)
Treatment refractoriness
Intermittency of treatment? (i.e., drug holidays may be an *increased* risk factor for persistent dyskinesia)

Recommendations: Since literature is overwhelmingly positive that maintenance on neuroleptic treatment prevents relapses in schizophrenics, consider long-term treatment (in nonbipolars who demonstrate a requirement for neuroleptics) with low to moderate doses (i.e., close to the minimal effective dose).

Assess risk-benefit ratios in relationship to:
  Diagnosis and available treatments
  Risks of treatment and of no treatment

roleptics themselves in the etiopathogenesis of tardive dyskinesia remains an area of some argument. A final liability of the neuroleptics is their proclivity to produce physical and subjective side effects that can be extremely dysphoric. Many patients suffer severe akathisia from these compounds as well as parkinsonian slowing and rigidity. The possibility also exists that the neuroleptics themselves interfere with reward systems in the brain and adversely affect motivation and possibly lead to depressive-like side effects.

Thus, there has been an intensive search for alternative and adjunctive treatments, which, to date, has only been partially successful. One of the more promising avenues of investigation involves the use of neuroleptics with some selectivity for blocking dopamine receptors in mesolimbic and mesocortical systems thought to be more intimately involved with psychotic processes, leaving dopamine receptors in the striatum (more directly linked to parkinsonian side effects) unaffected. An example of such a drug is clozapine which is now involved in systematic clinical trials in Europe and the United States and promises to be not only a compound with fewer extrapyramidal side effects, but potentially helpful in a subgroup of previously unresponsive schizophrenic patients. This drug has the liability of producing a hypo- or agranulocytopenia in as many as 10% of patients and requires close monitoring. The drug is available only on an investigational basis at the current time. Other drugs with similar selectivities are being sought, as well as partial dopamine agonists which could have preferential effects on presynaptic receptors and thus decrease dopaminergic function by increasing inhibitory tone.

Recent neuroscience advances in elucidating mechanisms involved in the biochemical actions of phencyclidine (PCP) also promise to provide a new generation of antipsychotic compounds. It has recently been discovered that glutamate and glycine are agonists that bind at the entry of calcium channels, with PCP binding at a site within the channel. Sigma opiates which can also increase psychosis bind at this or a closely related site. Thus, the psychotogenic properties of PCP, which can produce a clinical state highly similar to schizophrenia, are thought to be modulated through the effects on this ion channel. It is hoped that compounds acting directly at the PCP receptor or anticonvulsants active at glutamate receptors could thus ameliorate some psychoses that are more closely modeled by PCP and do not directly involve a primary lesion of dopaminergic mechanisms. Although no glutamate antagonist is currently available, it is of some interest that the anticonvulsant carbamazepine has been recently reported to decrease release of excitatory amino acids in the brain such as aspartate which may act on ion channels similar to glutamate.

ADJUNCTIVE STRATEGIES

Lithium Carbonate

Various approaches to supplementing neuroleptic treatment are summarized in Table 8-1. A clinical trial of lithium carbonate clearly deserves consideration in light of data suggesting that lithium alone in selected patients can be an important antipsychotic treatment even in schizoaffective and schizophrenic patients. Although it has been suggested that an increased growth hormone response to apomorphine may be associated with a good response to lithium in schizophrenia, clinical or biological markers indicating which patients might respond to this treatment used alone or as an adjunct are not readily available. Thus, it would appear useful for the refractory acute patient and the patient with chronic relapses to undergo a clinical trial with lithium. When the drug is effective it appears to target not only symptoms of overactivity and emotional dysregulation, but also some of the primary symptoms of the schizophrenic process, including thought disorder. Although it was initially hoped that cotreatment with lithium would prevent the development of neuroleptic-induced side effects based on its ability to block behavioral supersensitivity following chronic neuroleptic treatment in animals, clinical data in this regard have not been substantial. Nonetheless, on the basis of the excellent antipsychotic effects of lithium in some patients, a clinical trial in refractory schizophrenia would appear indicated.

Carbamazepine

A series of anticonvulsant compounds have emerged as important adjunctive treatments to the neuroleptics in some schizophrenic patients. Again the anticonvulsant carbamazepine leads the list of treatments in this category both on the basis of how extensively it has been studied and on the weight of the evidence derived from these studies. In uncontrolled studies, moderate or marked clinical efficacy has been reported with carbamazepine as an adjunct in 111 of 182 schizoaffective and schizophrenic patients (61%). More impressively, a series of 12 double-blind clinical case reports and trials are now available which document parallel findings. In most instances, carbamazepine when compared with placebo has been added to previously ineffective or only partially effective neuroleptic treatments. These studies demonstrate a consistent statistically significant and clinically relevant advantage for carbamazepine when compared with placebo. Moderate to marked responses occurred in 68 of 146 schizoaffective or schizophrenic patients (47%).

The primary symptoms targeted by carbamazepine appear to be those most affected in patients with manic-depressive illness including the excited phase of psychoses with grandiosity, emotional over- and underreactivity, conceptual disorganization, and aggression. However, in some instances, hallucinatory phenomena and primary thought disorders are also positively affected. As reviewed in Chapter 9, a highly consistent finding in both the open and controlled studies is that carbamazepine, as an adjunct to neuroleptics, may help in the treatment of hostility, aggression, and violence associated with the psychotic process. Scattered case reports

Table 8-4. Interactions Between Carbamazepine and Other Drugs

Influence of other drugs on carbamazepine levels	
Increased levels associated with toxicity	Increased levels without toxicity
Erythromycin	Valproate
Troleandomycin	(Carbamazepine-10,11-epoxide only)
Triacetyloleandomycin	Propoxyphene
Verapamil	Nicotinamide
Diltiazem (not nifedipine)	Cimetidine (mild acute increases, none
Isoniazid (not tranylcypromine)	after 1 week)
Viloxazine	
Nafimidone	Decreased levels
Danazol	Phenobarbital
	Phenytoin
	Primidone
	Theophylline

Influence of carbamazepine on other drugs	
Carbamazepine increases	Carbamazepine decreases
Escape from dexamethasone	Clonazepam
suppression	Dicumarol
Desmethylclomipramine	Doxycycline
Clomipramine	Valproate
Phenytoin	Theophylline
	Ethosuximide
	Warfarin
	Haloperidol
	Pregnancy tests

also suggest that it may be helpful with catatonic symptoms and in some instances may positively affect hallucinations.

Double-blind studies reporting the positive effects of carbamazepine as a neuroleptic adjunct have been conducted throughout the world including South Africa, Israel, Germany, and Japan. There are only isolated reports of exacerbation of psychosis with carbamazepine adjunctive treatment. Notable exacerbations have not been reported in controlled studies and these isolated case reports might be attributable to one of several factors. Initiation of carbamazepine treatment with too high a dose at the onset can sometimes produce behaviorally toxic side effects. Thus, it is recommended to begin with 200–400 mg/day rather than starting with 800 mg/day. High doses may also be associated with hyponatremia in rare instances. Finally, a series of studies has demonstrated that carbamazepine can markedly decrease plasma levels of haloperidol as much as 50%. Therefore, the isolated reports of exacerbation could be attributable to this factor as well. However, from the opposite perspective, the clinical improvement achieved with carbamazepine addition to neuroleptics may be even more remarkable as many of the studies utilized haloperidol as the neuroleptic in the primary treatment. Thus, the significantly greater degree of clinical improvement that was achieved by carbamazepine compared with placebo, occurred in the face of substantially reduced haloperidol levels. This represents one of several interactions of clinical relevance in this direction, and, as previously summarized on page 78 of Chapter 4, many different pharmacological agents can markedly increase carbamazepine levels leading to potential toxicity, and patients should be so warned. These include the macrolide antibiotics (e.g., erythromycin and troleandomycin), isoniazid, calcium channel blockers, verapamil and diltiazem (but not nifedipine), and viloxazine, nafimidine, and danazol (Table 8-4).

In a recent series examining the antipsychotic effects of carbamazepine, several patients who did not show any notable clinical improvement demonstrated marked exacerbations upon discontinuing carbamazepine therapy. The investigators postulated an atypical withdrawal syndrome that could be evident on carbamazepine discontinuation. The potential mechanisms for this clinical effect are not at all clear as carbamazepine has not been demonstrated to produce a substantial withdrawal syndrome following termination of therapy for epilepsy, trigeminal neuralgia, or affective illness. On the contrary, it is typical for treated symptoms to reemerge to the extent that they had previously occurred, and in the case of epilepsy, for some persistent anticonvulsant effects to be manifested in some clinical populations and in some animal models, such as aluminum cream cortical foci. Nonetheless, one should be aware of this potential danger in the discontinuation phase of carbamazepine in nonresponders treated for psychosis. In our series of depressed patients, some 50% of them were nonresponders and no evidence of withdrawal syndrome was observed. In addition, in the carbamazepine-antidepressant responders, there was little evidence for reemergence of depression upon drug discontinuation in contrast to the findings in mania where, following the second day of placebo substitution, manic symptoms often began to reemerge. As noted in the studies of Okuma and colleagues, it appears that the incidence of clinical response to carbamazepine progressively declines as one moves along the continuum from pure manic syndromes to schizoaffective to pure schizophrenic.

Valproate

Although valproate has demonstrated considerable promise as the second anticonvulsant behind carbamazepine in the treatment of bipolar illness, results do not appear to be quite as promising for this agent in the treatment of schizoaffective and schizophrenic patients. Whereas valproic acid may be effective in the treatment of some schizoaffective patients, the incidence of response in schizophrenic patients is quite low. Although this has not been systematically studied, presumably the levels of valproate targeted for potentiation would be in the same range as that observed in epilepsy (i.e., between 50 and 100 μg/ml). Clearly, further clinical and systematic controlled evaluation of the utility of valproate in schizoaffective and schizophrenic syndromes is warranted to better delineate its range of clinical efficacy.

Use of carbamazepine and valproate in combination has not been systematically explored in nonepileptic populations, although there is some clinical experience with the combination in epilepsy. However, there do appear to be isolated case reports of patients responding to the combination treatment, although it is not always clear whether there has been well-documented nonresponse to either agent alone. Moreover, when the two drugs are used in combination, valproate displaces carbamazepine from its protein-binding sites and may be associated with increases in side effects. Moreover, two cases of marked asterixis with isolated hyperammonemia and normal indices of liver function have been observed when the two drugs are used in combination.

Benzodiazepines

Benzodiazepine anticonvulsants have been utilized as adjuncts to neuroleptics with mixed results. A series of clinical reports notes at times dramatic amelioration of catatonic symptoms, hallucinosis, or moderate improvement in all aspects of the psychotic syndrome when high potency benzodiazepines (i.e., those with anticonvulsant efficacy) are added to existing neuroleptic treatment. Two double-blind studies have utilized alprazolam as an adjunct: one study reported statistically and clinically significant degrees of clinical improvement, whereas the other study showed negative results. Given the primary antipanic effects of alprazolam and clonazepam, a clinical trial of these agents might be placed at a higher level in the treatment hierarchy in the schizophrenic patient with high levels of anxiety and/or panic.

Clonazepam can be relatively sedating. However, this agent might be particularly useful for the patient with insomnia associated with his acute psychosis, perhaps with greater use as a nighttime sedative than a daytime maintenance treatment. Moreover, the benzodiazepine agents as a class are associated with the development of tolerance to their anticonvulsant efficacy, and whether this would also occur to their psychotropic effects for anxiety and for adjunctive treatment of psychosis remains to be further delineated, especially because most of the clinical trials to date have involved rather short-term courses of treatment.

Phenytoin

Phenytoin (Dilantin) has been widely promulgated in the lay press as a potential treatment agent for patients with acute and chronic schizophrenia as well as a variety of other psychiatric disorders. However, much of this literature is based on that collected many decades ago before systematic clinical trials using double-blind designs were fashionable. Therefore, the overall degree of antipsychotic efficacy of phenytoin as an adjunctive agent and in comparison to the other anticonvulsants remains an issue that requires further careful systematic clinical documentation. One fulminant psychotic patient with apparent schizoaffective illness was reported to show marked degrees of clinical improvement during four instances of treatment with phenytoin and exacerbation upon withdrawal on each occasion. This kind of clinical evidence in one patient suggests that other patients may also be responsive to this anticonvulsant. Perhaps a clinical trial with this anticonvulsant could be considered in the otherwise treatment refractory schizophrenic patient, particularly if other clinical approaches have been unsuccessful.

Acetazolamide

Acetazolamide (Diamox) is a carbonic anhydrase inhibitor anticonvulsant which has preliminarily been reported to have utility in the treatment of some isolated atypical psychoses. In particular, it has been reported in a Japanese trial that this anticonvulsant was effective in the treatment of patients with atypical confusional psychosis associated with dreamy states and also in those associated with puerperal or menstrual exacerbation. It is noteworthy that patients in this series appeared to respond to acetazolamide when they did not respond to the anticonvulsant carbamazepine or to the psychotropic agent lithium carbonate. Investigators in the United States have also suggested the utility of acetazolamide in combination with B6 in the treatment of some schizophrenic patients. It would appear that this compound is deserving of isolated clinical trials in the refractory patient, as well as more systematic double-blind clinical evaluation.

DIFFERENTIAL RESPONSE TO ANTICONVULSANTS?

From the very sparse data that are available in patients with psychiatric illness and the convergent data in patients with epilepsy, it would appear that some patients respond to one anticonvulsant agent when they do not respond to another. As discussed in Chapter 7, a schizoaffective patient responded to carbamazepine but not to phenytoin and valproate (see Fig. 7-12). Conversely, patients with severe psychotic manias who respond to valproate acutely and prophylactically when they do not to carbamazepine have been seen (see Fig. 7-11). Several cases in the literature suggest responses to clonazepam, alprazolam, lorazepam, or phenytoin. Taken together, these data would suggest a clinical strategy of rotating clinical trials in a sequential fashion in the neuroleptic nonresponder or partial responder, in the hopes that treatment response can be optimized.

Obviously, this strategy remains provisional until further systematic clinical data are available and the possible clinical or biological markers of treatment response are elucidated. However, given the relative absence of evidence that patients respond substantially better to one neuroleptic than to another (although the side-effect profiles and patient acceptability may differ markedly), consideration of adjunctive treatment with non-neuroleptic agents such as lithium and the anticonvulsants may be given higher priority than it was only a decade ago.

Given the vagaries of fluctuations in the clinical course associated with schizoaffective and schizophrenic syndromes, the psychopharmacologist would do well to develop clinical strategies for systematically following the acute and chronic course of the illness. In this regard, the construction of a life chart for the schizophrenic patient in a fashion similar to that suggested for patients with the affective disorders (see p. 148) is recommended. Instead of plotting manic and depressive episodes, one might plot positive and negative symptoms of the illness as well as a degree of functional incapacity. In this way the longitudinal prospective can be used in the evaluation of the efficacy of previous psychotropic treatments as well as current manipulations that are being attempted. In this regard the role of supportive measures based on regular physician contact as well as attempts at building more structured social support systems and aiding families in the management of what is often a devastating medical illness is emphasized. Recent data have supported a role for family intervention not only in its own right, but in relationship to a consistent emerging body of data indicating that excess degrees of expressed emotions in families may adversely impact on psychopathology and relapse in schizophrenic patients.

Viewed in this fashion, the anticonvulsants become a potential helpful adjunct to a variety of other therapeutic modalities in the approach to the acute and chronically psychotic patient. It would appear important to balance the hopeful perspective that one of these adjunct treatments may be of clinical benefit to the patient without overpromising a "cure" which appears to be extremely unlikely, even based on isolated anecdotal case reports. Nonetheless, improvement may be substantial in various areas of symptom reduction that can be of considerable benefit to the patient and his family. In particular, in relationship to the potential for aggressivity and violence, as documented in Chapter 2, a clinical trial of the anticonvulsants would appear to gain additional support in the overall assessment of the risk-to-benefit ratio and potential for clinically significant pharmacotherapeutic interventions.

SUGGESTED READING

Carpenter WT, Heinrichs DW, Hanlon TE. A comparative trial of pharmacologic strategies in schizophrenia. *Am J Psychiatry* 1987;144:1466–1470.

Dalby MA. Behavioral effects of carbamazepine. In: Penry JK, Daly DD, eds. *Complex Partial Seizures and Their Treatment (Advances in Neurology,* vol 11). New York: Raven Press, 1975:331–343.

DeVeaugh-Geiss J, ed. *Tardive Dyskinesia and Related Involuntary Movement Disorders.* Boston: John Wright-PSG, Inc., 1982.

Dose M, Apelt S, Emrich HM. Carbamazepine as an adjunct of antipsychotic therapy. *Psychiatr Res* 1987;22:303–310.

Folks DG, King LD, Dowdy SB, Petrie WM, Jack RA, Koomen JC, Swenson BR, Edwards P. Carbamazepine treatment of selected affectively disordered inpatients. *Am J Psychiatry* 1982;139:115–117.

Hakola HPA, Laulumaa VAO. Carbamazepine in violent schizophrenia. In:Emrich HM, Okuma T, Muller AA, eds. *Anticonvulsants in Affective Disorders.* Amsterdam: Excerpta Medica, 1982:204–207.

Kalinowsky LB, Putnam TJ. Attempts at treatment of schizophrenia and other non-epileptic psychoses with Dilantin. *Arch Neurol Psychiatry* 1943;49:414–420.

Kidron R, Averbuch I, Klein E, Belmaker RH. Carbamazepine-induced reduction of blood levels of haloperidol in chronic schizophrenia. *Biol Psychiatry* 1985;20:199–228.

Klein E, Bental E, Lerer B, Belmaker RH. Carbamazepine and haloperidol vs. placebo and haloperidol in excited psychoses. *Arch Gen Psychiatry* 1984;41:165–170.

Kubanek JL, Rowell RC. The use of Dilantin in the treatment of psychotic patients unresponsive to other treatment. *Dis Nerv Syst* 1946;7:47–50.

Lambert PA. Acute and prophylactic therapies of patients with affective disorders using valpromide (dipropylacetamide). In: Emrich HM, Okuma T, Muller AA, eds. *Anticonvulsants in Affective Disorders.* Amsterdam: Excerpta Medica, 1984;33–44.

Lautin A, Angrist B, Stanley M, Gershon S, Heckl K, Karobath M. Sodium valproate in schizophrenia: some biochemical correlates. *Br J Psychiatry* 1980; 137:240–244.

McElroy SL, Keck PE Jr, Pope HG Jr. Sodium valproate: its use in primary psychiatric disorders. *J Clin Psychopharm* 1987;7:16–24.

Post RM, Uhde TW. Anticonvulsants in non-epileptic psychosis. In: Trimble MR, Bolwig TG, eds. *Aspects of Epilepsy and Psychiatry.* Chichester, England: John Wiley & Sons, 1986:177–211.

Post RM, Uhde TW, Joffe RT, Bierer L. Psychiatric manifestations and implications of seizure disorders. In: Extein I, Gold M, eds. *Medical Mimics of Psychiatric Disorders.* Washington, D.C.: American Psychiatric Association Press, 1986:35–91.

Puzynski S, Klosiewicz L. Valproic acid amide in the treatment of affective and schizoaffective disorders. *J Affect Disord* 1984;6:115–121.

Stramek J, Herrera J, Costa J, Heh C, Tran-Johnson T, Simpson G. A carbamazepine trial in chronic, treatment-refractory schizophrenia. *Am J Psychiatry* 1988;145:748–750.

Stevens JR, Bigelow L, Denney D, Lipkin J, Livermore A, Rauscher F, Wyatt RJ. Telemetered EEG-EOG during psychotic behaviors of schizophrenia. *Arch Gen Psychiatry* 1979;36:251–262.

Takezaki H, Hanaoka M. The use of carbamazepine (Tegretol) in the control of manic-depressive psychosis and other manic-depressive states. *Clin Psychiatry* 1971;13:173–183.

Wolkowitz OM, Breier A, Doran A, Kelsoe J, Lucas P, Paul SM, Pickar D. Alprazolam augmentation of the antipsychotic effects of fluphenazine in schizophrenic patients. *Arch Gen Psychiatry* 1988;45:664–671.

Wyatt RJ, Alexander RC, Egan MF, Kirch DG. Schizophrenia, just the facts. What do we know, how well do we know it? *Schizophrenia Res* 1988;1:3–18.

9

Anticonvulsants in the Treatment of Aggression and Dyscontrol

Robert M. Post

RELATIONSHIP OF SEIZURES TO DYSCONTROL

The relationship of dyscontrol to epilepsy is extremely controversial. Although numerous case reports and courtroom dramas have depicted the occurrence of violent acts during the ictal process, recent large collaborative studies, using simultaneous EEG recordings and videotapes in patients prescreened for dyscontrol acts, failed to show a substantial relationship between these phenomena. Thus, it would appear that at best, aggressive acts carried out during a seizure are extremely rare.

Nonetheless, many ambiguities arise in determining the precise relationship between interictal irritability, aggression, and violence and their relationship to complex partial seizures or other seizure types. Again, although case reports and selected studies suggest an increased incidence of aggression and dyscontrol in the context of complex partial seizures, broader-based epidemiological approaches indicate that such problems are extremely rare. The complex relationship between seizures and aggressive behavior may be illustrated by several different types of animal models of limbic epilepsy. Repeated administration of subconvulsant doses of local anesthetics, such as lidocaine, eventually produce an increase in physiological responsivity which results in the occurrence of major motor seizures (a pharmacological kindling phenomenon).

Electrical Kindling

In 1969, Goddard and associates first described the phenomenon of electrophysiological kindling, where repeated stimulation of the amygdala (e.g., once a day for 1 second) would result in a lowering of the afterdischarge threshold; increasing duration, spread, and complexity of afterdischarge; and a progression of seizure stages, finally culminating in the appearance of major motor seizures involving tonic-clonic movements of head, trunk, and forepaws with rearing and falling. Once the animals were kindled in this fashion, they remained permanently susceptible to seizure induction even 6 months to a year after kindling had ceased. Moreover, if seizures were repeatedly induced, a stage of spontaneity could be reached during which animals would demonstrate seizures in the absence of electrophysiological stimulation.

A similar progression appears to occur with the local anesthetics including the emergence of spontaneous seizures. The lidocaine seizures are behaviorally similar to those achieved by amygdala kindling and involve increases in metabolic activity in amygdala, hippocampus, or perirhinal cortex associated with electrophysiological spiking in the amygdala. Lidocaine seizures increase the rapidity of electrophysiological kindling, and electrical kindling increases the incidence of lidocaine seizures, further suggesting that the two share common substrates. However, the behavioral consequences of the two seizures are markedly different.

Local Anesthetic Kindling

Although initial studies reported some increases in irritability and "resistance to capture" in animals kindled from the amygdala and the hippocampus (but not the caudate nucleus), subsequent reports by many other investigators have failed to document this finding. Amygdala-kindled animals, aside from a brief period of postictal hyperactivity, do not show noteworthy changes in basal aggressivity toward conspecifics (other rats) or the experimenter. In contrast, animals repeatedly given lidocaine seizures show marked changes in aggressivity. In particular, if the animals are housed in isolation, directed attacks toward animal handlers may occur upon opening of the cage. When animals are housed together, occasionally they are found with tails eaten off or the other animal eaten. However, it is particularly noteworthy that this aggression does not occur during the seizure episode or even in the immediate postictal period, but is clearly an interictal phenomenon which appears to predispose the animal toward aggressive responding for a period of some days to weeks after the lidocaine seizures. In this instance the lidocaine seizure is a clear model for interictal aggressivity. The induction of the seizure is required, as animals pretreated with equal doses of lidocaine, which do not experience seizures, do not show this aggressivity. In contrast, Adamec, working with cats that were natural killers of rats, observed that stimulation of the amygdala to lower the after-discharge threshold (but short of the induction of major motor seizures), would be sufficient to convert these animals into nonkillers. Thus, these observations stress the importance of stimulation characteristics and species differences in responses to kindling stimuli; responses differ markedly depending on electrophysiological versus chemical-kindling induction.

Peptides

Consideration of a last model of chemical-induced aggression may further serve to highlight these principles. A single dose of corticotropin-releasing factor (CRF) administered into the ventricles can produce spiking in the amygdala and the onset of limbic seizures some 4 to 8 hours after injection. These seizures appear behaviorally identical to those achieved by amygdala or lidocaine kindling. Yet the behavioral consequences are quite different. In contrast to lidocaine-kindled animals, which demonstrate aggression particularly toward an outside experimenter, animals receiving CRF may engage in vicious attacks against conspecifics. Moreover, this may occur in the absence of a seizure or immediately in the interictal period between convulsive episodes. Thus, the type, time-course, patterning, and the directiveness of the aggression all appear to vary considerably in animals displaying three different types of seizure induction (electrical, lidocaine, CRF) which produce virtually identical behavior seizures.

Environmental Context

A last preclinical observation is of importance to the clinical discussion of the relationship of epilepsy to aggressive behavior. It has been repeatedly observed that the environmental context is critical to the behavioral consequences of brain stimulation. Identical characteristics of brain stimulation can have virtually opposite behavioral consequences depending on the context. For example, if a cat with an electrode in the thalamus is stimulated while it is in a place associated with food and water, it will purr contentedly. In contrast, if it receives the same stimulation characteristics through the same electrode while it is in a place where it has previously received electrical shock, it will demonstrate a rage reaction. Similar differences in responsivity have also been demonstrated for hypothalamic placements. Moreover, animals will perform considerable amounts of work in order to receive a brain stimulation reward, indicating that it obviously has considerable positive consequences. Yet, if the same electrical currents are administered through the same electrode by the experimenter (i.e., the animal does not bar press for the delivery of current), the stimulation will be adversive. These findings highlight the importance of environment context, behavioral state, volitional control, and related psychosocial variables that can profoundly affect the behavioral response to altered electrophysiological activity.

ANTICONVULSANTS FOR DYSCONTROL

Given this ambiguous, multifaceted, and complex relationship of preictal, ictal, and interictal activity to episodes of aggression, it is understandable that a clear relationship among EEG abnormalities, aggressive behavior, and response to the antiaggressive effects of anticonvulsants has not emerged. In fact, the data across a number of studies suggest that patients both with and without EEG abnormalities may show antiaggressive responses to the use of anticonvulsant agents (Luchins, 1983,1984).

Although the anticonvulsants as a class of drugs appear to have considerable use in the treatment of dyscontrol, it is important to note that response to one anticonvulsant may not predict response to another. This clinical suggestion is based on not only case vignettes, but also a considerable experimental literature indicating that different anticonvulsant agents may be differentially effective in different animal models of aggression. No clinical study has demonstrated adequate predictors of response to the range of antiaggressive agents or to individual compounds within the anticonvulsant series. Thus, in the absence of such empirical data, how might the clinician proceed?

Diagnostic Evaluation: Treatment of the Underlying Illness

Psychiatric Syndromes

A useful clinical principle would appear to be that treatment of the aggressive individual ought to proceed with a careful diagnostic evaluation and therapeutic approaches toward adequate treatment of the primary psychiatric or medical diagnosis. Thus, if violence and aggression are emerging as concomitants of a manic episode, approaches to aggression and violence should be directed at the treatment of the underlying manic-depressive illness and may include the use of lithium carbonate, anticonvulsants, and neuroleptics as discussed in detail in Chapter 7. Similarly, aggression emerging in the context of a schizophrenic episode or in a patient with epilepsy should be initially focused on the treatment of these underlying disorders. In these instances, initial diagnostic approaches may critically impact on choice of pharmacotherapy. For example, the diagnosis of multiple personality disorder, which can often present with episodes of extreme rage, would direct one toward the use of psychotherapy, hypnotherapy, and related psychological approaches given the absence of data suggesting anything more than transient clinical responses to a variety of psychotropic agents in the treatment of this syndrome. The diagnosis of multiple personality disorder should be considered in the patient presenting with a complex variety of symptoms that may span a variety of diagnostic categories and be associated with bizarre episodic behavior, a history of time lapses or amnesia, headaches, atypical auditory hallucinosis, depression, insomnia, and sudden behavioral changes.

Drug Abuse

Similarly, very different therapeutic prescriptions are given for the patients with violence in the context of drug abuse. Therapeutic work aimed at abstinence for the alcoholic, particularly with the use of support groups such as Alcoholics Anonymous, may be critical to the success of the treatment, and in many instances, may be more important than pharmacotherapeutic approaches. Cocaine and phencyclidine (PCP) should also be considered in relationship to possible drug precipitants of aggressive behavior. Violent acts can often occur in the cocaine user in the context of extreme paranoia. Cocaine in this regard appears to present the dual liabilities of amphetamine-like catecholaminergic stimulation as well as a pure local anesthetic with its proclivity for inducing anxiety, irritability, and limbic seizures. Violent episodes in the PCP abuser may be grotesque and catastrophic with manifestations of extreme strength, imperviousness to pain, and indiscriminant mutilation of even close associates, friends, and relatives. During a PCP episode, usual tactics of "talking a patient down" are ineffective, and seclusion with prolonged monitoring for possible recrudescence of violence is indicated. Opinion is mixed regarding the utility of haloperidol for PCP-induced psychosis and dyscontrol, and agents which specifically work at the PCP receptor (which modulates calcium channels) along with glutamate, glycine, and magnesium are eagerly awaited. Presumably, the next generation of anticonvulsant agents, which act as glutamate antagonists, may play a role in the treatment of PCP psychosis, although this proposition has its theoretical ambiguities and remains to be directly clinically tested. Endogenous ligands for the PCP receptor have been isolated and again it may be hoped that specific blockers of this site may be effective in the treatment of PCP intoxication. It is problematic that agents such as MK-801, which exert anticonvulsant and antistroke potential in animal models, appear to be psychotogenic. Perhaps the more specific glutamate antagonists, such as AP5 or AP7, will emerge as clinically effective anticonvulsants with a positive spectrum of behavioral effects.

Although treatment of the violent cocaine abuser has not been adequately elucidated, several clinical trends appear to be emerging. Desipramine has been demonstrated in double-blind studies to be more effective than lithium or placebo in reducing cocaine-induced craving. Dopaminergic agonists such as bromocriptine also hold promise based on clinical and preclinical data. Specific programs to decondition stimuli which provoke craving, abstinence reactions, or conditioned euphoria and related psychological approaches focused on supporting abstinence also appear critical.

Preclinical data by Post and Weiss (1988) also suggest a possible role for the anticonvulsant carbamazepine in selected circumstances of cocaine intoxication. However, it should be emphasized at the onset of this discussion that controlled trials have not been performed to demonstrate this postulated role, and there are considerable liabilities involved. Whereas chronic oral carbamazepine blocks the development of lidocaine- and cocaine-kindled seizures in our animal model in the rat, it should be noted that an acute dose of carbamazepine may actually exacerbate cocaine-induced seizures and their associated lethality. Thus, if there is a role for the anticonvulsant carbamazepine in the treatment of cocaine-related phenomena, it must be a highly delineated one, reserved for the patient able and willing to assume a clinical trail of chronic administration, not with the illusion that carbamazepine would provide acute coverage or an antidote for a cocaine-related episode or seizure. Carbamazepine does not block catecholamine receptors and does not block acute cocaine- or amphetamine-induced hyperactivity. Moreover, it does not block the increased behavioral responsivity to cocaine demonstrated on repeated administration (behavioral sensitization). In man, treatment with carbamazepine also does not block stimulant-induced euphoria with methylphenidate. Thus, carbamazepine may or may not be able to block the psychomotor-stimulant properties of cocaine, but appears capable of blocking to its local anesthetic effects. Preliminary data suggest that some patients with cocaine-related panic attacks may show adequate response to the anticonvulsants carbamazepine and clonazepam, where they do not show adequate responses to more typical agents for panic such as the tricyclic antidepressants. Given the wide range of studies suggesting the utility of carbamazepine across a variety of diagnostic entities in the treatment of aggressive patients, the use of carbamazepine might be considered in the violent cocaine user, particularly if there is a history of cocaine-related seizures or panic attacks. If there is a prominent component of paranoia, neuroleptic treatment would appear appropriate.

Borderline Personality Disorder

Aggressivity and violence in the context of borderline personality disorder deserves special attention for several reasons. First, the study of Cowdry and Gardner (1988) represents the best controlled study of multiple medications in this disorder yet to be performed, and the theme of the interrelationships of aggression, impulsivity, and aggression directed toward the self (suicidal behavior) is particularly well illustrated. In this study, 16 female outpatients with borderline personality disorder and prominent behavioral dyscontrol were included in a double-blind cross-over trial of placebo to four active medications including alprazolam (average dose, 4.7 mg/day); carbamazepine (average dose, 820 mg/day); trifluoperazine hydrochloride (Stelazine, average dose, 7.8 mg/day); and tranylcypromine sulfate (Parnate, average dose, 40 mg/day). In terms of the overall clinical effects, there was considerable discrepancy between physician and self-ratings. Physicians rated carbamazepine and tranylcypromine significantly better than placebo. However, patients rated themselves significantly improved relative to placebo only while receiving tranylcypromine.

There was a marked dysjunction in the effects of medications on the behavioral dyscontrol. During the placebo period there were six patients with moderate and two with severe dyscontrol. During alprazolam treatment, this increased to one moderate and eight severe episodes such that the clinical trial had to be discontinued. During carbamazepine treatment, there were no severe and only one moderate episode, a highly statistically significant improvement. There were no significant changes with the other agents.

The episodes of dyscontrol in this patient population during alprazolam administration were not trivial; they included assaults, severe wrist-cutting, and slashing of the neck. These data illustrate the importance of considering anticonvulsants as a nonunitary class. Alprazolam is an anticonvulsant with considerable potency at the benzodiazepine receptor. However, in this report of Cowdry and Gardner and in other instances in the clinical literature, benzodiazepines have been reported to paradoxically facilitate aggressive behavior and induce dyscontrol episodes. In contrast, another anticonvulsant, carbamazepine, which appears to exert its effects not through the central-type benzodiazepine receptor, but through the so-called peripheral-type, showed clear superiority among the other psychotropic and anticonvulsant agents and in comparison to placebo in inhibiting impulsive and dyscontrol acts. Although the patients' subjective sense of dysphoria did not improve significantly during carbamazepine treatment, physicians' ratings of clinical improvement in depression, impulsivity, and suicidality were clearly improved with this agent (Fig. 9-1).

Systematic clinical trials of other anticonvulsants in the treatment of patients with borderline personality disorder remain to be conducted, but preliminary data suggest that some patients may also respond to ethosuximide. The utility of valproate and phenytoin (which has been widely touted for use in other syndromes) clearly deserves careful clinical trials.

Nonetheless, the early clinical data suggest a clear advantage of carbamazepine over several other categories of psychotropic drugs (monoamine oxidase inhibitors and neuroleptics) in the treatment of dyscontrol acts in borderline personality disorders and a relative contraindication for the anticonvulsant alprazolam in this patient population. Do the differences in these two anticonvulsants arise from their differential anticonvulsant efficacy on peripheral-type versus central-type benzodiazepine receptors or some other mechanism of action of carbamazepine? This question

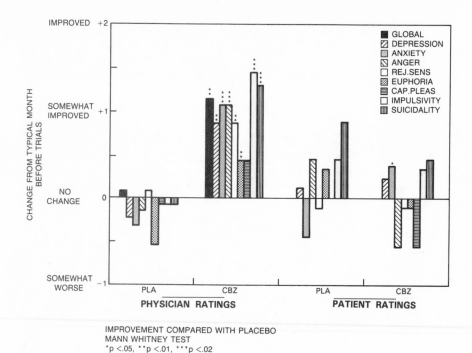

FIG. 9-1. Differential impact of carbamazepine on physician-versus-patient ratings. PLA, placebo. Redrawn from Gardner and Cowdry (1988) with permission.

remains for further preclinical and clinical exploration but the possibility also arises that other unique effects of carbamazepine that account for its psychotropic properties as distinct from its anticonvulsant effects may be important in this regard.

Aggression, Impulsivity, Suicidal Behavior: Relationship to Low Serotonin

Studies of Brown, Goodwin and colleagues (1986) at the NIMH not only demonstrate the interrelationships among aggression, impulsivity, and suicidal behavior, they suggest that these three factors may have a common relationship to low serotonin as measured by the serotonin metabolite 5-hydroxyindoleacetic acid (5-HIAA) concentrations in the cerebrospinal fluid (CSF) of patients with personality and conduct disorders studied at the Bethesda Naval Clinic. These investigators found a significant inverse correlation between CSF 5-HIAA and a lifetime history of aggressive acts, a variety of measures of impulsivity, as well as ratings of suicidal ideas and impulses. The findings of low 5-HIAA in relation to suicidal behavior appear to be consistent across a variety of patient diagnoses, and such relationships have been observed in patients with depression (unipolar only), schizophrenia, and a variety of personality disorders.

Data in animals and man suggest that manipulation of serotonergic tone by serotonin precursors or giving diets deficient in tryptophan may respectively ameliorate or exacerbate hostility or aggression. Thus, it is of interest that carbamazepine, in contrast to phenytoin and phenobarbital, increases plasma tryptophan (i.e., a precursor of brain serotonin). Thus, it is possible that effects of carbamazepine on serotonergic mechanisms or other effects not directly attributed to its anticonvulsant properties could account for its broad range of effects on aggressive syndromes and other of its psychotropic properties. This proposition clearly remains to be directly tested, but would predict the greater efficacy of carbamazepine compared with phenytoin in dyscontrol syndromes where low serotonin may be etiologically important.

Choice of Anticonvulsants

When carbamazepine is administered as an adjunct to neuroleptics in either opened or controlled studies compared to placebo in the treatment of schizophrenic patients, positive effects not only on psychotic but also aggressive symptoms have been reported in the literature with few exceptions. In most studies, the findings have been both statistically significant and clinically robust. In several studies, dramatic clinical remissions have been observed in selected patients, such as in violent schizophrenic women with years of incarceration who have been able to be discharged from the hospital following adjunctive treatment with carbamazepine. Thus, based on both the controlled clinical trials demonstrating a statistical advantage of carbamazepine over placebo, as well as open clinical studies and case vignettes, it is recommended that the adjunctive use of carbamazepine in the violent schizophrenic patient be considered relatively early in the sequence of clinical trials.

Again, it is important to emphasize that although some of these patients have been chosen for EEG abnormalities, those selected for the absence of EEG abnormalities have shown an equal degree and incidence of positive antiaggressive effects to the addition of carbamazepine. In one study, carbamazepine reduced numbers of aggressive acts compared with base line and when carbamazepine was discontinued for administrative reasons, an increased frequency of aggressive acts was observed; patients improved again when carbamazepine was reinstituted. Thus, in addition to controlled clinical trials, such "off-on-off-on" observations further document a role for carbamazepine in decreasing numbers of aggressive acts in patients across a variety of diagnostic entities.

Beta-blocking drugs, such as propranolol, have been widely used in the treatment of aggression. However, at recommended doses (up to 800 mg/

day), it is very unlikely that beta-blocking effects are selective, and at these high doses, propranolol has been considered "membrane stabilizing," if not anticonvulsant. In support of this view are the findings in mania that high doses of both *d* and *l* isomers are therapeutically effective even though only one isomer effectively blocks beta receptors. Nonetheless, this treatment along with lithium deserves high consideration among the nonanticonvulsant approaches to the treatment of aggression and dyscontrol. Propranolol should be initiated at doses of 20 mg three times a day and increased by 60 mg every 3 days until a clinical response or a limit of 800 mg/day is achieved. Response may occur in a matter of days, but may require up to 8 weeks.

Although valproate may be effective in some animal models of aggression, not only are systematic clinical trials unavailable, but open studies and clinical vignettes are virtually absent from the literature. In contrast, considerable literature, mostly of an uncontrolled nature, exists for the anticonvulsant phenytoin. Given these ambiguities based on a lack of an empirical clinical data base, we would suggest that carbamazepine be utilized first in a series of anticonvulsants in attempts at primary or adjunctive treatment of the aggressive patient. Clearly, if there are other indicators such as the concomitant presence of spike and wave (generalized absence seizures) which can be exacerbated by carbamazepine, but are treated by valproate, a different order of drug treatment may be considered and instituted.

Carbamazepine (over phenytoin) is suggested not only because of the larger data base considering its utility in aggressive dyscontrol syndromes, but also in terms of its associated profile of positive psychotropic effects and its side-effect profiles. As reviewed in other chapters, carbamazepine appears capable of exerting positive effects on dysregulated mood, and to the extent that these factors may be contributing to dyscontrol, the drug may be helpful. In contrast, there is evidence, as reviewed in Chapter 2, that phenobarbital and phenytoin in some instances can be associated with increases in depression, dysphoria, or cognitive impairment in epileptic patients. As indicated above, the anticonvulsants clonazepam and alprazolam might be considered with a much lower priority for use in dyscontrol syndromes because of their potential for paradoxical induction of dyscontrol, as well as their potential for dependence and abuse liability.

If carbamazepine were to be used in sole or adjunctive treatment of dyscontrol syndromes, many of the principles elucidated for the use of this agent in the treatment of manic-depressive illness (see Chapter 7) would appear to apply. Slow increases in dose, titrated against individual side effect thresholds, would appear important in order to avoid typical anticonvulsant side effects and the associated potential for noncompliance. Dose-response relationships for treatment of aggressive syndromes have not been adequately delineated in clinical studies, such that titration to mild (and then away from) clinical side effects in order to achieve optimum doses and blood levels would appear a prudent way to proceed.

SUGGESTED READING

Brown GL, Goodwin FK. Human aggression: a biological perspective. In: Reid WH, Dorr D, Walker JI, Bonner JW, eds. *Unmasking the Psychopath: Antisocial Personality and Related Syndromes*. New York: W. W. Norton and Co., 1986:132–155.

Cowdry RW, Gardner DL. Pharmacotherapy of borderline personality disorder. Alprazolam, carbamazepine, trifluoperazine, and tranylcypromine. *Arch Gen Psychiatry* 1988;45:111–119.

Gardner DL, Cowdry RW. Anticonvulsants and personality disorders. In: McElroy SL, Pope HG, eds. *Anticonvulsants in Psychiatry: Recent Advances*. Clifton, NJ: Oxford Health Care, 1988:127–140.

Lion JR, Tardiff. The long-term treatment of the violent patient. In: Hales RE, Frances AJ, eds. *Psychiatry Update: APA Annual Review*. Washington, DC: American Psychiatric Association Press, 1987:537–548.

Luchins DJ. Carbamazepine for the violent psychiatric patient. *Lancet* 1983;1:766.

Luchins DJ. Carbamazepine in violent non-epileptic schizophrenics. *Psychopharmacol Bull* 1984;20:569–571.

Mattes JA. Carbamazepine for uncontrolled rage outbursts. *Lancet* 1984;2:1164–1165.

Mattes JA, Rosenberg MS, Mays D. Carbamazepine versus propranolol in patients with uncontrolled rage outbursts: a random assignment study. *Psychopharmacol Bull* 1984;20:98–100.

Monroe RR. Anticonvulsants in the treatment of aggression. *J Nerv Ment Dis* 1975;160:119–126.

Monroe RR. Limbic ictus and atypical psychosis. *J Nerv Ment Dis* 1982;170:711–716.

Neppe VM. Carbamazepine as adjunctive treatment in nonepileptic chronic inpatients with EEG temporal lobe abnormalities. *J Clin Psychiatry* 1983;44:236–331.

Post RM. Lidocaine kindled limbic seizures: behavioral implications. In: Wada JA, ed. *Kindling 2*. New York: Raven Press, 1981:149–160.

Post RM. Behavioral effects of kindling. In: Parsonage M, ed. *Advances in Epileptology: XIVth Epilepsy International Symposium*. New York: Raven Press, 1983;173–180.

Post RM, Weiss SRB. Psychomotor stimulant versus local anesthetic effects of cocaine: role of behavioral sensitization and kindling. In: *Mechanisms of Cocaine Abuse and Toxicity*. Washington, DC: U.S. Government Printing Office, NIDA Research Monograph 88, 1988:217–238.

Sheard MH. Clinical pharmacology of aggressive behavior. *Clin Neuropharmacol* 1984;7:173–183.

Tunks ER, Dermer SW. Carbamazepine in the dyscontrol syndrome associated with limbic system dysfunction. *J Nerv Ment Dis* 1977;164:56–63.

Index

A

Acetaminophen, 80,83
Acetazolamide, 92
  manic-depressive illness, 144
  and primidone, 79
  schizophrenia, 154,161
N-Acetylprocainamide, 62
α_1-Acid-glycoprotein, 58–59
Acidosis, 94
S-Adenosylmethionine, 29
Affective disorders in epilepsy, 28–30,34; see also Manic-depressive (bipolar affective) illness; Schizophrenia/schizoaffective disorders, neuroleptic with adjunct anticonvulsant treatment
Age, 64
Aggression, 24
Aggression/dyscontrol, anticonvulsant treatment, 165–175
  carbamazepine, 173,174
  environmental context, 167
  neuroleptics, 168,173
  peptides, 167
  propranolol, 173–174
  seizures and, 165–167
  serotonin, low levels, 172–173
  underlying illness, treatment, 168–172
    borderline personality disorder, 170–172
    drug abuse, 169,170
    manic-depressive illness, lithium, 168,174
    personality disorders, 168,173
    schizophrenia, 168,173
  valproate, 174
Agonists and inverse agonists, 141
Agoraphobia, 31
Albumin, drug plasma binding, 56–60
Alcohol abuse, 169
  withdrawal seizures, 35–37

Alcoholic epilepsy, 35
Alkalosis, 94
Allopurinol and phenytoin, 76
Alprazolam, 170,171
  manic-depressive illness, 120,123, 142–144
  schizophrenia, 154,160,162
Alzheimer's disease, 21
Amiodarone, 55,76
Amitryptyline, 30
  pharmacokinetics, 69
Amoxapine, pharmacokinetics, 69
Amygdala, 19,20
  kindled seizures, manic-depressive illness, 133–135,141–142,144–146
Androgens and carbamazepine, 78
Antacids and antiepileptics, 76,78–79
Antibiotics, 63,66; see also specific antibiotics
Anticoagulants and phenytoin, 77
Antidepressants, 30
  heterocyclic, 120,122–123
  tricyclic, 2,58,59,69,96,120,122–124,144,145
  see also specific drugs
Antiepileptic/anticonvulsant drugs, 10–11
  and cognitive functioning, 11–14
  children, 106–110
  EEG, 37–39
  pharmacodynamics, 89–97
    historical background, 89–90
    mechanism of action, 90–96
    psychiatric drugs, 96–97
  side-effects, 11–15
  see also Aggression/dyscontrol, anticonvulsant treatment; specific disorders and drugs
Antiepileptic/anticonvulsant drugs, interactions, 71–87
  cognitive function, 71

Antiepileptic/anticonvulsant drugs, interactions (*cont'd*)
  drug absorption, 78–80
  drug–drug interactions, 72,74–78
    carbamazepine, 78
    liver enzymes, 74–77,82–87
    phenobarbital, 79
    phenytoin, 76–77
    primidone, 79
    protein binding displacement, 75–76,82
    valproic acid, 78
  generic drugs, 81–82
  idiosyncratic interactions, 72–74
  kinetics, zero-order (saturation), 72
  metabolism
    autoinduction, 82–84
    induced by other drugs, 84–85
  rashes, 73
Antipyrine, 80
Anxiety
  childhood, 106
  in epilepsy, 21,29,31
Attention-deficit hyperactivity disorder, childhood, anticonvulsants for, 99–104,109
Attention impairment, antiepileptics/anticonvulsants, 37,38
Auras, 4
Autism, 21
Automatisms, 5

B
Barbiturates, 27,28,30; *see also specific drugs*
Beck's Depression Inventory, 107
Behavior disorders. *See* Childhood, behavior disorders
Behavioral toxicity, antiepileptic/anticonvulsant drugs, 14
Bipolar affective disorder. *See* Manic-depressive (bipolar affective) illness
Borderline personality, 170–172
Bromocriptine, 120
BUN elevation, renal failure, 58
Buproprion, 120
Butyrophenones, 35,36

C
Calcium channel blockers, 120,146, 154; *see also specific drugs*

Carbamazepine, 6,10,11–15,38,39, 75–76,91–93,96
  ADHD, 101–102,110
  aggression/dyscontrol, 173,174
  alcohol withdrawal seizures, 36–37
  alteration of other drugs, listed, 80
  borderline personality, 170–172
  cimetidine, 74
  cf. clonazepam, 142,143
  cocaine interaction, 170
  and cognitive function, 107–110
  conduct disorder, 105,106,110
  drug interactions, 78,158
  erythromycin and, 74,76
  generic, 81
    and nongeneric, 78
  inhibition by other drugs, 85
  manic-depressive illness, 114–124
    cf. lithium, 114–116,119–121, 124–132,147
    prophylaxis, 131–136
  mechanism of action, 93–95
  pharmacokinetics, 68
  and phenytoin, 77
  and primidone, 79
  psychiatric problems in epilepsy, 27,29–30
  schizophrenia, 154,157–159,161, 162
  cf. valproate, 78,138–141
  see also under Manic-depressive (bipolar affective) illness
Carbamazepine 10,11-epoxide, 84, 109,158
Carbonic anhydrase inhibitors, 79
Caucasians, 64
CGS-8216, 142
Childhood, behavior disorders, 99–110
  ADHD, 99–104,109
  anticonvulsants and cognitive function, 106–110
  anxiety disorders, 106
  conduct disorder, 103–106,109
Children's Depression Inventory, 106–107,109
Chloral hydrate and phenytoin, 77
Chloramphenicol, 77,80
Chloripramine, 120
Chlorpromazine, 2,35,77,78
Chromatography, 42
Cimetidine, 80,86
  and carbamazepine, 74,78,158
  phenytoin, 74,77

Classification, epilepsy, 7–8
    and psychiatric problems, 22
    cf. seizures, 1
Clobazam, 10–14,31
    ADHD, 103,110
    alcohol withdrawal seizures, 36
    cognitive effects, 39
Clomipramine, 30,158
Clonazepam, 10–12,14,80,92
    ADHD, 102,110
    anxiety disorders, childhood, 106
    and carbamazepine, 158
    cognitive effects, 39
    manic-depressive illness, 120,139,
        141–144
    schizophrenia, 154,160,162
Clorazepate, 92
Clozapine, 156
Cocaine, 169,170
Cognitive functioning
    and antiepileptics/anticonvulsants,
        11–14,21,71
    in children, 106–110
    EEG, 37–39
Conduct disorder, childhood, anticon-
    vulsants for, 103–106,109
    diagnostic criteria, 104
Congestive heart failure, 63
Connors Parent Symptom Question-
    naire, 106,107
Contraceptives, oral, 15,80
Control. *See* Aggression/dyscontrol,
    anticonvulsant treatment
Coumadin and phenytoin, 77
Cursive seizures, 5
Cyclosporine, 80

D

Danazol and carbamazepine, 78,
    158,159
Delusions, 154,160
Dementia and epilepsy, 21
Deoxycycline, 80,158
Depression
    in epilepsy, 21,22,28,29,30
    seizures, classifications, 5,6
    see also Manic-depressive (bipolar af-
        fective) illness
Desimpramine, pharmacokinetics, 69
Desmethylclomipramine, 158
Dexamethasone, 80,158
Diabetes insipidus, 124
Diazepam, 103

alcohol withdrawal seizures, 36
    manic-depressive illness, 142
Diazoxide and phenytoin, 77
Dicumarol, 77,80,158
Digitoxin, 80
Diltiazem, 78,158,159
Dipropylacetamide, 136
Disulfiram and phenytoin, 77
Dopamine metabolism, schizophrenia,
    153
Dosage interval, 67
Dosage regimens, 41,45–46
Doxepin, pharmacokinetics, 69
Drug absorption, 55–57
    drug interactions, 78–80
Drug abuse, 169,170
Drug metabolism, 60–62
    drug interactions, 84–85
    genetic factors, 61,63–64
DSM-III, 147
DSM-IIIR, 20,21,99–101,103,106
Dyscontrol. *See* Aggression/dyscontrol,
    anticonvulsant treatment
Dysthymic disorder, 28–30

E

Electroconvulsive therapy (ECT),
    30,35,113–114,120
Electroencephalography (EEG)
    aggression/dyscontrol, 168,173
    antiepileptics/anticonvulsants, cog-
        nitive functioning, 37–39
    attention-deficit hyperactivity disor-
        der, childhood, 102
    conduct disorder, childhood, 105
    manic-depressive (bipolar affective)
        illness, 118,121,122,141
    psychiatric problems in epilepsy, 19–
        21,23–25,32,35
    seizure classifications, 2–4,6,7
    valproic acid, 94
Encephalopathy, insidious, 39
Environmental context, aggression/
    dyscontrol, 167
Enzyme immunoassay technique
    (EMIT), 42
Epilepsy, 1,7–15
    alcoholic, 35
    causes, 8–10
        listed, 9
    classification, 7–8
        cf. seizures, 1
    historical view, 17,18

Epilepsy (*cont'd*)
  psychiatric problems. *See* Psychiatric
    problems in epilepsy
  reflex, 9
  see also Seizures
Erythromycin
  and carbamazepine, 74,76,78,158,
    159
  and phenytoin, 74
Eskimos, 64
Ethosuximide, 10,14,92,171
  and carbamazepine, 158
  cognitive effects, 39
  mechanism of action, 95–96
  pharmacokinetics, 68

F
Fear, 22,32
Fetal hydantoin syndrome, 129
Flunarizine, 146
Fluoxethine, pharmacokinetics, 69
Folic acid, 29,77

G
GABA, 91,94,95,145–146
GABA receptor, 141,145
Gelastic seizures, 5
Generalized seizures, 3–4,6,10,11,91,
    92
Generic drugs, interactions with non-
    generics, 81–82
Genetics, drug metabolism, 61,63–64
Geschwind syndrome, 24
Glucuronic acid, 60
Griseofulvin, 80

H
Half-life, 51–52,54
Hallucinations, 2,5,7,154,160
Haloperidol, 35,80,101,155,158,159
Hepatitis, 62
Hepatotoxicity, valproic acid, 73,74
5-HIAA, 172
Hippocampus, 19,20
Historical view, epilepsy, 17,18
HVA, 153
Hydantoin, fetal, syndrome, 129
Hydroxylation, phenytoin, 60–62,69,83
Hypergraphia, 24,25–28

Hyponatremia, 128
Hyposexuality, 24–25

I
Ibuprofen and phenytoin, 77
Imipramine, 30,69
Individual variations, pharmacology,
    43,46,55–63
Intelligence quotient, anticonvulsants
    and, children, 107
Iprindole, 96
Isoniazid, 87
  and carbamazepine, 78,158
  and phenytoin, 77
  and primidone, 79

J
Japanese, 64

K
Kluver-Bucy syndrome, 20

L
Lennox-Gastaut syndrome, 8,21,102
Lidocaine, 59,80,166,167
Lithium, 14,94,96–97
  schizophrenia, 154,156–157
  vs. valproate, 137,138
Liver microsomal enzymes, drug me-
    tabolism, 60,61,74–77,86,87
Lorazepam, 36,162
Loxapine and phenytoin, 77

M
Macrolide, 86
Magnetic resonance imaging, 34
Manic-depressive (bipolar affective)
    illness, 96–97,113–150,159
  acetazolamide, 144
  amygdala-kindled seizures, 133–
    135,141–142,144–146
  calcium channel blockers, 120,146
  carbamazepine, 114–124
    acute depression, 118–124
    acute mania, 114–118,119,121
    blood levels, 117–118
    cf. neuroleptics, 115,116,120,130

prophylaxis, 131–136
rash, 128–129
response predictors, 116
sleep, 117
cf. unipolar depression, 118–120
carbamazepine vs. lithium, 114–116,119–121,124–132,147
diabetes insipidus, 124
potentiation, 122,124,126,131–132
pregnancy, 130
side-effects, hematologic, 125–127
thyroid hormones, 125,127–128,131–132
clonazepam, 120,139,141–144
EEG, 118,121,122,141
electroconvulsive therapy, 113–114, 120
in epilepsy, 28
GABA, 145–146
graphic depiction, life-course of illness, 146–150
lithium, 168,174
phenytoin, 139,140,144–145
cf. carbamazepine, 144–145
treatment sequences, 120
valproate, 120,129,136–141
vs. carbamazepine, 138–141
Maprotiline, 2,30,69
Methsuximide, 92
Methylphenidate and phenytoin, 77
Metoprolol, 80
Metronidazole and phenytoin, 77
Mianserin, 2,30,96
Miconazole and phenytoin, 77
Minimum effective concentration, 67
Minimum toxic concentration, 67
Minnesota Multiphasic Personality Inventory, 19,23,32
MK-801, 169
Monoamine oxidase inhibitors, 120,123,124,131,132,143,144, 146
Mono- vs. polytherapy, 37–38
Myocardial infarction, 58–59
Myoclonic seizures, 3,5,10,11,92

N
Nafimidone, 158,159
National Institute of Mental Health, 115,118,131,132
Neuralgia, trigeminal, 114,133,145, 159

Neuroleptics
aggression/dyscontrol, 168,173
discontinuation, 137
extrapyramidal side-effects, 155
parkinsonism, 155,156
tardive dyskinesia, 116,154–156
manic-depressive illness, 115,116, 120,130
vs. valproate, 137
see also Schizophrenia/schizoaffective disorders, neuroleptic with adjunct anticonvulsant treatment; specific drugs
Nicotinamide, 78,79,158
Nirvanol, 82
Nitrazepam, 11
Nitrofurantoin and phenytoin, 77
Noncompliance, recognition, 45,63
Nortriptyline, 69,72,80

O
Oral contraceptives, 15,80
Orosomucoid, 58–59

P
Pancreatitis, acute, 73,74
Panic attacks, 31,106
Paranoid schizophrenia, 6–7
cf. in epilepsy, 32–35
Parkinsonism and neuroleptics, 155,156
Partial seizures, 2,4–7,10,11,91,92, 95,121
Personality disorders
and epilepsy, 21,23–24
multiple, 168,173
Pethidine, 80
Petit mal seizures, 4
Pharmacodynamics, 46–49; see also under Antiepileptic/anticonvulsant drugs
Pharmacology, 41–69
dosage interval, 67
dosage regimens, 41,45–46
drug absorption, 55–57
drug metabolism, 60–62
genetic factors, 61,63–64
drug utilization altered by disease, 43–44,58–59,62
individual variations, 43,46,55–63
noncompliance, recognition, 45,63
patient information, 64–66

Pharmacology (*cont'd*)
  pharmacodynamics, 46–49
  pharmacokinetics, 49–55
    half-life, 51–52,54
    kinetics, 50–51,52,59
    single dose, fate, 52–53
    steady state, 53–55
    zero-order, 72
  physiologic states, changing, 45,
    57–58
  plasma protein binding and free drug
    concentrations, 56–60
  renal excretion, 62–63
  steady-state concentrations, moni-
    toring, 67–69
  therapeutic drug monitoring, 41–
    46,64
Phenacemide, 77,79
Phencyclidine (PCP), 156,169
Phenobarbital, 71,79,80,83,90,92,173
  and carbamazepine, 78,158
  mechanism of action, 95
  pharmacokinetics, 68
  and phenytoin, 77,80
Phenobarbitone, 10,11,14,15
  ADHD, childhood, 101,102,110
  cognitive effects, 39,109,110
  conduct disorder, 104–106
  psychiatric problems in epilepsy,
    29,30
Phenothiazines, 2,35,36,77,78
Phenylbutazone, 77,80
Phenytoin, 10–15,38,39,71,72,91,92,
  171,173,174
  alcohol withdrawal seizures, 36
  alteration of other drugs, 80
  antiepileptic drugs, interactions, 76–
    77
  and benzodiazepines, 77
  and carbamazepine, 158
  childhood, 110
  cimetidine, 74,77
  discovery, 90
  erythromycin, 74
  fast and slow preparations, 81
  generic, interactions with nonge-
    neric, 77
  hydroxylation, 60–62,69,83
  manic-depressive illness,
    139,140,144–145
  mechanism of action, 93,95
  pharmacokinetics, 68
  phenobarbital, 80
  and primidone, 79,80

psychiatric problems in epilepsy, 30
schizophrenia, 154,161,162
and valproate, 60,69,75,82
P-450 enzymes, 74,75,82–85
Phobias in epilepsy, 31
Pimozine, 35
Pleasure centers, 20
Polytherapy
  cognitive function, children, 107–
    109
  vs. monotherapy, 37–38
Positron emission tomography, 34
Potassium bromides, 89–90
Prednisolone, 80
Pregnancy
  manic-depressive illness, 130
  tests, carbamazepine and, 158
Primidone, 10,54,65,91,92
  alteration of other drugs, 80
  antiepileptic drugs, interactions, 79
  and carbamazepine, 78,158
  childhood, 110
  generic, 79,81
  half-life, 65
  mechanism of action, 95
  pharmacokinetics, 68
  phenytoin, 80
Procainamide, 59,62,64
Prodromata, 4
Propoxyphene, 86–87
  and carbamazepine, 78,158
  and phenobarbital, 79
  and phenytoin, 77
Propranolol, 80
  aggression/dyscontrol, 173–174
  schizophrenia, 154
Protein-binding displacement, drug
  interactions, 75–76,82
  valproic acid, 75,82
Protein binding, plasma, and free drug
  concentrations, 56–60
Protriptyline, pharmacokinetics, 69
Pseudoseizures, 10
Psychiatric problems in epilepsy, 17–
  35
  anxiety, 21,29,31
  carbamazepine, 27,29–30
  classification, 22
  cognitive dulling, 21
  dementia, 21
  depression, 21,22,28,29,30
  EEG, 19–21,23,24,25,32,35
  electroconvulsive therapy, 30,35
  fear, 22,32

ictally related disorders, 21–23
interictal disorders, 23–35
  affective disorders, 28–30,34
  aggression, 24
  hypergraphia, 24,25–28
  hyposexuality, 24–25
  psychoses, 31–35
  religiosity, 24,25,27
  suicide, 28
manic-depressive psychosis, 28
panic attacks, 31
cf. paranoid schizophrenia, 32–35
personality disorders, 21,23–24
phenobarbitone, 29,30
phenytoin, 30
phobias, 31
psychoses and, 31–35
temporal lobe epilepsy, 18–20, 24,25,28,31–33
Psychogenic seizures, 9–10
Pyridoxine and, 77,79,80

Q
Quinidine, 59

R
Radioimmunoassay, 42
Rash, drug, 73,128–129
Receptor pharmacodynamics, 46–49
Reflex epilepsy, 9
Religiosity, 24,25,27
Renal excretion, pharmacology, 62–63
Renal failure, BUN elevation, 58
Rifampin, 77,79
Ro5-4864, 142
Ro15-1788, 142

S
Salicylates, 77,78,80,83
Schizophrenia, 168,173
  paranoid, 6–7
  cf. epilepsy, 32–35
Schizophrenia/schizoaffective disorders, neuroleptic with adjunct anticonvulsant treatment, 155–163
  acetazolamide, 154,161
  alprazolam, 154,160,162
  calcium channel blockers, 154
  carbamazepine, 154,157–159,161, 162

  clonazepam, 154,160,162
  delusions, 154,160
  differential responses, 161–163
  dopamine metabolism, 153
  hallucinations, 154,160
  lithium, 154,156–157
  phenytoin, 154,161,162
  propranolol, 154
  valproate, 154,159–162
Seizures
  in aggression/dyscontrol, 165–167
  alcohol withdrawal, 35–37
  auras, 4
  automatisms, 5
  cases, 6–7
  classifications, 1–7
  cursive, 5
  depression, 5,6
  EEG changes, 2–4,6,7
  gelastic, 5
  generalized, 3–4,6,10,11,91,92
  hallucinations, 2,5,7
  listed, 2
  myoclonic, 3,5,10,11,92
  partial, 2,4–7,10,11,91,92,95,121
  petit mal, 4
  prodromata, 4
  pseudoseizures, 10
  psychogenic, 9–10
  threshold, drugs lowering, 2,35
  tonic–clonic, 3,92
Serotonin in aggression/dyscontrol, 172–173
Sleep, 117
Spina bifida, valproic acid, 129
Spironolactone, 120
Status epilepticus, 5–6
Steady-state concentrations, 53–55,67–69
Stevens-Johnson syndrome, 129
Substance P, 94
Succinimides and phenytoin, 77
Sucralfate and phenytoin, 77
Suicide/suicidal behavior, 28,172–173
Sulfonamides and phenytoin, 77
Sulthiame, 10

T
Tardive dyskinesia, 116,154–156
Temporal lobe epilepsy, 17,18–20,24,25,28,31–33
Theophylline, 66,72,80,158

Therapeutic drug monitoring, 41–46,64
Thioridazine, 77,101
Thyroid hormones, 80,125,127–128, 131–132
Tonic–clonic seizures, 3,92
Tranylcypromine, 171
Trazodone, pharmacokinetics, 69
Triaceyloleandomycin, 158
Trifluoperazine hydrochloride, 170–171
Trigeminal neuralgia, 114,133,145, 159
Troleandomycin, 78,158,159
Tryptophan, 120,136,173

U

Unipolar cf. bipolar depression, 118–120
Uremia, 63
U.S. Food and Drug Administration, 81,90

V

Valproate/valproic acid, 10–14,91–93,171

aggression/dyscontrol, 174
antimania, 120,129,136–141
    vs. carbamazepine, 138–141
and carbamazepine, 138–141
and cognitive function, 39,107–110
conduct disorder, childhood, 105
generic and nongeneric, 78,81
half-life, 54,65
hepatotoxicity, 73,74
interactions, 78
mechanism of action, 94–95
pancreatitis, acute, 73,74
pharmacokinetics, 68
and phenobarbital, 79
and phenytoin, 60,69,75,82
protein-binding displacement, 75,82
schizophrenia, 154,159–162
spina bifida, 129
Verapamil, 78,158,159
Viloxazine, 158,159

W
Warfarin, 80,158
Weight, patient, 64–65
West's syndrome, 8